D1252279

PATHOLOGY
for
Funeral Service

1st Edition

Published by

PROFESSIONAL TRAINING SCHOOLS, INC.
4722 Bronze Way   Dallas, Texas 75236

i

Table of Contents

Chapter One
INTRODUCTION TO GENERAL PATHOLOGY

Pathology may be defined as the study of disease - specifically, the study of the structure and function of the body as it is affected by disease. The term pathology comes from the Greek word for disease or suffering (pathos), and the word for science, or the "study of" (logos). Therefore, we can see that pathology is intimately related to the fields of anatomy and physiology, which are concerned with the normal structure and function of the human body. When structure and function are no longer "normal", the field of pathology comes into play.

Centuries ago the practice of medicine, including the study of disease, fell within the field of religion, and was practiced by priests and other religious figures. In these early times, it was believed that diseases affecting mankind were the result of super-natural powers and spirits. It was the job of religious leaders to chase these evil spirits away, and hopefully, rid the body of disease. With advancing civilization, much practical knowledge was accumulated, experiments were performed, and observations were made, all of which led to a gradual movement away from supernatural beliefs in the field of medicine to a more natural understanding of events and occurrences.

The ancient Egyptians and Greeks did much to advance the study of medicine and disease, with one particular Greek physician named Hippocrates (460-359 B.C.) contributing a great many theories and advances. The teachings of Hippocrates were so widely acclaimed that he is often credited with being the "Father of Medicine", and the Hippocratic oath professed by modern day physicians is based on his ideas of honor and ethical practice of the medical profession.

Over the centuries, many changes and discoveries in the fields of anatomy and bacteriology improved medical practices and the ability of doctors to successfully operate on and treat their patients. In the early 1800's, a German professor of pathology by the name of Rudolph Virchow made significant contributions to the field by elaborating his theories on the cellular basis of disease. Previous to his discoveries, physicians understood that the body was sick, or individual areas or organs were diseased, but did not relate these problems to the individual cells making up these tissues and organs. Virchow explained the concept that all disease resulted primarily from changes adversely affecting the cells of the body. He is therefore often referred to as the "Father of Cellular Pathology".

The overall field of pathology is often broken down into several subdivisions as follows:

1) **Gross Pathology** - studies changes in the structure and function of the body which can be observed with the unaided eye.

2) **Microscopic, Cellular, or Histo-Pathology** - studies changes which occur in cells of the body at the microscopic level. The use of a microscope is required for this aspect of pathology.

3) **General Pathology** - deals with general or broad disease processes, such as necrosis or inflammation, which may affect the entire body or widespread tissues and organs.

4) **Special Pathology** - studies disease processes affecting individual body areas or systems, such as pathology of the respiratory system or diseases of the skin.

5) **Pathological Anatomy** - deals with the study of tissues which have been removed from the body for pathological study. If they were removed during surgery, as a biopsy, it may be referred to as surgical pathology, or if removed during autopsy, it would be called autopsy pathology.

6) **Clinical Pathology** - deals with the laboratory study of, and the performance of standardized tests on, body fluids and secretions, such as blood and urine tests, or cultures and smears of various types.

7) **Physiological Pathology** - refers to studying the functional changes in the body resulting from disease.

8) **Medical-legal Pathology (Forensic Pathology)** - that field of pathology which deals with both the medical and legal issues surrounding death.

The Autopsy

The term **autopsy,** from the Greek words for "self" and "sight", is used to refer to the examination of the body after death in order to determine the cause of death and/or the existence of various disease conditions. Two other terms which are often used synonymously with autopsy are **post-mortem examination,** from the Latin words for "after" and "death", and **necropsy,** from the Greek word for "a state of death".

The autopsy is an important part of the study of pathology, and has been used for centuries by physicians and scientists to learn more about the structure and function of the body as well as learning about pathological conditions. An autopsy involves both the gross examination of the human body and its organs and tissues, plus the microscopic examination of tissue samples and cells which have been removed for further study.

Following is a list of some important benefits which the autopsy provides to the medical and funeral professions:

1) It helps to confirm, or possibly alter, the medical diagnosis. By allowing a pathologist to closely view the body's tissues and organs, and to run auxillary tests, the autopsy may provide evidence to substantiate the original diagnosis. On the other hand, it may provide additional or new information which may significantly alter the doctor's original assumptions about death or disease in a particular case.

2) It contributes to medical knowledge. As a result of being able to perform autopsies, the medical profession has learned a great deal over the years about various diseases, how to treat them, and hopefully how to prevent their recurrence in the future.

3) It is valuable in medical-legal cases. The field of forensic pathology has made great strides over the years in assisting legal authorities concerning the cause of death in numerous types of situations, such as homocide, suicide, and accident cases.

4) It helps satisfy the minds of survivors about the cause of death and/or the existence of disease. This is of particular importance to the professional funeral director in his/her role as a caregiver and counselor when dealing with families. The autopsy can provide important evidence concerning the cause of death to family members or friends who are struggling emotionally with the loss of someone who is dear to them. Whether the evidence provided is what they wanted to hear or not, it nevertheless will

help them to see the reality of what has occurred, and hopefully assist in the psychological healing process which they will face.

A professional funeral director will maintain a positive and cooperative attitude toward the autopsy. When dealing with autopsied cases, and even when discussing the autopsy with those involved with a funeral service, the funeral director should exhibit a service-minded approach. He/she should always remember to speak tactfully and professionally when discussing the autopsy, whether it is with another professional in the medical field or a family member who is being served.

Disease

If we describe pathology as the study of disease, we should certainly have an understanding of what we mean by "disease". We can think of the term disease as being the opposite of health. Webster's dictionary defines health as "the condition of being sound in body, mind, or soul, especially freedom from disease or pain". Hence, when a body is healthy, disease is not present, and when disease is present, a body is not healthy. Certainly there are great variations in the nature and severity of diseases, from those which are very minor to those which are serious and even fatal.

Literally, the word disease is a combination of the prefix "dis" meaning "to free of" or "undo", and the word "ease", meaning a state of well being or lack of pain. Based on this literal meaning, we can understand that disease is in fact the "undoing of a state of well-being." Possibly a more practical definition when studying the field of pathology is to describe **disease** as any change in the structure or function of the body as a result of injury to the tissues.

There are many descriptive terms which are used in the study of disease, such as those indicating how widespread a disease is, how rapidly it develops, how serious it is, what some of its characteristics are, etc. For example, the term **acute** describes a disease with a relatively rapid onset and short duration, whereas **chronic** refers to a disease with a slower onset and a generally longer duration. Exact time frames cannot be assigned to these terms, but a mention of some common examples may help to understand their usage. We all know that a common cold seems to come upon us rather suddenly, and usually lasts for only a short period of time, such as several days to a week or so. On the contrary, most cancers take a long time to develop within the human body, and usually last for extended periods of time - months or years. In this scenario, a cold could be described as an acute disease, and cancer as a chronic one. In addition, acute diseases may develop into chronic ones if they tend to recur with unusual regularity, or begin to persist over longer than normal time periods. An acute disease which is particularly severe and sudden in its onset, and often proves fatal, is called a **fulminating** disease.

The term **recurrent,** meaning to come back, or recur, is used to describe diseases which show alternating increases and decreases in their symptoms. **Infectious** diseases are those caused by pathogenic microorganisms, and **contagious** or diseases are those which are easily transmitted from person to person. **Infestation** refers to the presence of macroscopic (visible to the unaided eye) organisms in or on the body, such as animal parasites. Sometimes the cause of a disease is not known, in which case it may be called an **idiopathic** disease. When a disease results from the nature of one's working conditions, it is referred to as an **occupational** disease.

Other terms are used to describe how often, or when, a disease occurs, or how widespread it is at a given time. For instance, **endemic** diseases are those which are always present to some degree in a given area or community, while **sporadic** diseases are those which are found to occur only occasionally in a community. **Epidemic** refers to diseases which affect a much larger than normal number of people in a community at one time, and **pandemic** diseases are those which affect the majority of the population in a very large area, possibly even world-wide. Another way to describe a pandemic disease is one which is epidemic in many different parts of the world at the same time. **Prevalance** refers to the number of cases of a disease within a certain population at a given time. The term **acquired** is often used to categorize any disease which was obtained after birth, as opposed to **congenital** diseases, which are those present at birth. If a disease results from the fact that a person inherited some sort of abnormal genes from his/her parents, it may be called an **hereditary** disease.

Some of the characteristics exhibited by various diseases also lead to the use of terminology reflecting these characteristics. **Febrile** diseases are characterized by fever, **intoxicating** diseases by the presence of poisons or other toxic substances, and **deficiency** diseases are characterized by the lack of some essential dietary ingredient. An **iatrogenic** disease is one which results from a physicians treatment of a patient.

Another major category of diseases is referred to as **malformations** or **anomalies.** These conditions can be described as any defect in formation, structure, or position of a body part. Malformations can result from many causes, such as inheriting abnormal genes and chromosomes, which may result in defective development, or even absence, of a given body part. Chemical agents, such as drugs or poisons, which enter the system of a pregnant woman, may also result in serious developmental problems. Medical history books, as well as our current day health care system, are full of examples of babies being born with serious problems as a result of maternal drug or alcohol abuse. Other factors such as trauma to an unborn child, excessive radiation, or living agents such as bacteria and viruses, may lead to numerous malformations. Examples include birth defects which commonly result from a pregnant woman being infected with the bacteria which causes syphilis, or the virus causing rubella, also known as German measles. Some estimates place the likelihood of a child being born with a birth defect as high as 50% if a mother contracts German measles during the first month of pregnancy.

Examples of malformations or anomalies include the following:

1) **aplasia** - absence of a body part; amelia is a form of aplasia in which one or more limbs is missing.

2) **hypoplasia** - under development of a body part; phocomelia is a form of hypoplasia, in which the proximal portions of the extremities are absent or poorly formed.

3) **spina bifida** - a defect in the walls of the lower part of the spinal columnn, where the bones do not form properly, and may result in a protrusion of the spinal cord and membranes out of the spinal cavity. It is often referred to as a congenital fissure of the spinal column. (*See Fig. 1*)

4) **polydactylism** - an excess number of fingers or toes.

5) **hernia** - protrusion of an organ through the wall of the body cavity in which it is contained. (*See Fig. 2*)

6) **fistula** - an abnormal tract or channel through the tissues, connecting one body cavity with another, or connecting a cavity with the surface of the body.

7) **cyst** - a sac-like structure, containing fluid or a semi-solid substance. Usually results from the abnormal development of tissues, obstruction of ducts, or infections.

8) **Down's Syndrome (Mongolism)** - genetic defect resulting in various degrees of mental retardation, a dwarfed physique, and certain characteristic abnormalities of the head and extremities.

In addition to these types of diseases, other important terminology must be understood before proceeding into a more detailed study of pathology. Also, it must be remembered that disease was described as any change in the normal structure and function of the cells in the body, and it is difficult to separate the discussion of altered structure and altered function. It is not hard to imagine, for instance, that if the structure of a cell is significantly altered, it will unlikely be able to perform its normal function in a proper manner.

Structural changes produced in the tissues as a result of disease are referred to as **lesions.** Many diseases, called **organic** diseases, have readily identifiable, characteristic lesions associated with them, such as the swollen and inflamed mucous membranes of strep throat, or characteristic ulcerations present during syphilis. Others, called **functional** diseases, have no such characteristic lesions when they occur, such as migraine headaches or various mental disturbances called psychoses.

The term **symptom** is used to describe subjective indications of the presence of disease in the body. This means that the patient can experience something, such as pain, but it is not apparent or observable by the doctor. Examples of symptoms include itching, pain, nausea and dizziness. On the other hand, a **sign** is an objective indication of the presence of disease, such as fever or swelling, which can be observed by the doctor as well as being experienced by the patient. A **syndrome** is a group of symptoms or signs which usually appear together to indicate the presence of a particular disease. Doctors take symptoms and signs into consideration when making a **diagnosis,** which refers to the identification of a disease, and a **prognosis,** which is a prediction of the probable outcome of a disease.

Additional terms used to describe diseases include **remission** or **abatement,** which means that there has been a let-up in the severity of a disease, with diminished signs and symptoms. For example, cancers are often said to be in remission after various therapies have been employed on a patient, and the patient's condition seems to have improved. This does not mean that the disease has been cured, but only that it has significantly diminished for the time being. **Exacerbation** refers to a sudden increase in the severity of a disease, while a **complication** is any unfavorable condition which occurs during the course of a disease. An example of exacerbation might be a sudden increase in fever during a disease, likely indicating a turn for the worse in a patient's condition. A complication could be any number of circumstances occurring during a disease, such as hemorrhage accompanying stomach ulcers, or a patient contracting a secondary infection such as pneumonia while lying in a hospital bed being treated for a fractured hip.

Etiology

The term **etiology** refers to the study of the causes of disease. Closely associated with the cause of a disease is the manner in which it develops, or the various changes a disease goes through, resulting in damaged structure and function of the cells of the body. **Pathogenesis** is the term given to this manner of development of a disease. A doctor will take into consideration the pathogenesis of a disease when deciding how to best treat it and to come up with a prognosis.

One way to classify causative factors in disease is to determine whether or not a given factor actually caused a disease, or just made it more likely that a person would get the disease. Things which fall into this latter category, meaning they increase one's susceptibility to a disease, but don't actually cause it, are called **predisposing** factors. On the other hand, those things which actually do cause a disease are referred to as **exciting** or **immediate** factors. Following is a list of some common predisposing factors in disease:

1) **age** - being old or being young does not cause a disease, but age certainly predisposes toward various conditions. For example, heart and arterial diseases are much more common later in life, while infectious diseases such as measles, mumps, and chicken pox occur more frequently in the young. This has a lot to do with the development of the immune system, and the production of antibodies over the years. Children are more likely to develop many diseases because they have not built up immunities to the degree that an adult has been able to.

2) **race** - many studies over the years have concluded that people of different races have significant differences in their susceptibility to various diseases and resistance to others. A prime example is the fact that sickle-cell anemia is confined mostly to blacks, seldom affecting people of caucasian descent. On the contrary, blacks seem to be more resistant to such diseases as malaria and yellow fever. In addition, American Indians seem to be particularly susceptible to tuberculosis, and Jewish people fairly resistant to the disease.

3) **sex** - aside from the diseases associated with the reproductive organs, which only a person of one sex or the other would contract, women seem to be generally more resistant to diseases than men, with longer life spans to show for it. Another example is the inherited bleeding disorder called hemophilia, which is confined mostly to men.

4) **nutrition** - poor nutrition can lead to a generally weakened condition of the human body, making it more susceptible to various diseases. On the contrary, overeating can lead to obesity, which in turn predisposes to other disease conditions such as heart problems.

5) **occupation** - one's occupation may have an important bearing on their likelihood of obtaining a specific disease. A good example is the occupation of a coal miner. Due to their constant exposure to high levels of coal dust in the work environment, they are much more likely to contract anthracosis, or black lung disease, than someone in the general population.

6) **stress and emotion** - many studies over the years have shown that working and living under highly stressful or emotional conditions can weaken a person's resistance to disease and make it more likely that they succumb to various diseases which they might otherwise have avoided.

7) **environment** - one's living environment can predispose to various diseases. For example, people living in dark, damp, or overcrowded conditions may be predisposed to acquiring diseases which would not have affected them if their living conditions had been improved.

8) **economic status** - some authors like to discuss economic status as a separate predisposing factor in disease, while others consider it more of a general category encompassing several of the previously mentioned factors. For example, it may be argued that due to one's economic status, that person may experience more stress, live in a poorer environment, and be employed in occupations which are traditionally more dangerous, less safety conscious, etc.

As opposed to these predisposing factors in disease, many other factors can be described as immediate or exciting, meaning they are directly responsible for causing a disease, such as the following:

1) **living agents** - this includes various microorganisms, such as bacteria, viruses, and parasites, which are responsible for hundreds of infectious diseases affecting the human body.

2) **trauma** - trauma is from the Greek word for "wound", and is used to describe any physical injury to the tissues of the body, such as cuts, bruises, scrapes, or fractures.

3) **physical agents** - this category includes such factors as heat, cold, electricity, and radiation. When something hot burns the tissues, or freezing cold causes frostbite, we can say that these factors were directly responsible for the tissue injury which occurred. Likewise, electrical shock or excessive radiation, such as in sunburn, can cause significant damage to the body.

4) **chemical agents** - strong chemicals such as acids or alkalis can result in serious tissue destruction, as can various poisons or drugs taken into the body. Consequently, these chemical agents would be immediate factors, as they were responsible for the damage to the tissues.

5) **deficiencies** - many diseases are a result of the body's lack of some essential dietary item, such as a vitamin or mineral necessary for normal body function. A good example would be the disease called rickets, which can result from a diet lacking in vitamin D. Without vitamin D, the body cannot properly absorb calcium from the digestive tract, and calcium is needed for proper bone formation. This resulting lack of calcium can lead to soft and deformed bones. In addition to dietary deficiencies, various diseases result from deficiencies of important hormones normally present in the body. For example, too little pituitary growth hormone in a developing child can result in an abnormally small individual known as a dwarf. In each of these cases, the deficiency was the immediate factor in the disease, as the lack of this essential substance was directly responsible for the disease occurring.

6) **allergens** - allergens are foreign particles such as dusts or pollen, which are responsible for reactions occurring within the body of a person who is particularly sensitive to these allergens. An allergen which causes a reaction in one person may have no effect on another. When a given person has one of these abnormal reactions, they are said to be allergic to that substance. Consequently, an **allergy** can be described as a state of hypersensitivity to a foreign protein.

7) **heredity** - when the fertilization of an ovum occurs, beginning the process of a new life developing, a certain amount of genetic material is passed on

from both the father and mother of the new child. If one or more of the genes this child inherits are defective, the characteristic controlled by that gene is likely to be flawed. Many diseases known to science result directly from the inheritance of defective genetic material. Although heredity is often an immediate factor in disease, one's genetic make-up may also be a more general predisposing factor in certain diseases.

As we can see from our discussion so far, there is no easy answer to what causes many diseases. A doctor will have to consider many factors, predisposing and immediate, when trying to determine the cause of a particular disease. Although treatment of a disease does not necessarily require a thorough understanding of cause, it is certainly desireable to know as much as possible about the origin and development of a disease, and not just have to treat its symptoms and signs.

In continuing our study of general pathology, it will be helpful to further categorize the overall processes which occur in the body during disease. Included in this discussion will be such areas as circulatory disorders, metabolic disturbances and regressive tissue changes, inflammations, and neoplasms or tumors.

Chapter Two
Circulatory Disorders

The circulatory system in the human body includes the heart, which acts as the central pump, and an intricate arrangement of blood and lymph vessels which serve to transport blood and fluid throughout the body. Not only is the circulatory system responsible for delivering oxygen and nutrients to the cells of the body, but also for transporting waste products of cellular metabolism for eventual elimination. When something goes wrong with the process of circulation, the effects can be widespread and possibly disastrous. If these vital transportation functions are significantly altered, localized problems may occur, or generalized, widespread results may become evident. In this section we will discuss some of the general conditions which result from circulatory disturbances, and treatment of diseases affecting specific circulatory organs, such as the heart or blood vessels, will be undertaken later in the section on special pathology.

Hyperemia

Hyperemia, or **congestion,** is a condition which refers to excess blood in a body part. The term hyperemia is quite appropriate, as it comes from the prefix "hyper-", meaning excessive, and the suffix "-emia", which indicates a blood disorder. The term congestion is also used, indicating that blood is congested in a given part of the body. Just as traffic on our freeways becomes congested during rush hours, the blood in our circulatory system may also become congested at times. This may or may not be a good occurence, as will be discussed shortly. It should be pointed out that hyperemia does not mean that there is an excess of total blood volume in the body. It simply means that of the normal amount of blood present in your body, at any given time there may be an excess of this blood in a certain body part.

Hyperemia may result from the fact that there has been extra blood delivered to a body part, or that drainage of blood from an area has been impaired. This serves as the basis for dividing hyperemia into the two main categories of active and passive hyperemia.

Active hyperemia may be described as excess blood in a body part which was actively, or purposefully, taken there by the arterial system in the body. This increased blood flow to a body part may be further described as active **physiological** hyperemia if it results from a normal, everyday, healthful bodily function. Examples of this would be the presence of extra blood in the muscles of the body during exercise, as the need for extra oxygen is greatly increased during such activities. Also, in order to dissipate the heat generated from this greater muscular activity, there will be extra blood present in the skin, resulting in the common reddened face, or "flushed" appearance, of someone doing vigorous exercise. If active hyperemia is a result of some disease process, it would be termed active **pathological** hyperemia. For example, when tissues are injured and inflammation occurs, extra blood is delivered to the affected body part in an effort by the body to remedy the diseased condition and return the part to normal use. Contained within the blood are such things as platelets, white blood cells, and antibodies, all of which are involved in the body's internal protective mechanisms. During active hyperemia, the area is usually reddened, somewhat swollen, and warmer than normal. We will continue to discuss active pathological hyperemia in the section on inflammation.

Passive hyperemia occurs when venous drainage from an area is decreased.

There is extra blood in the area not as a result of the arteries delivering this extra blood there, but because blood cannot leave the area in normal fashion. Passive hyperemia is always pathological, and may be localized or generalized. When hyperemia is localized, it results from blockage of veins draining a particular area. The most common reasons for localized passive hyperemia to occur are as follows:

1) formation of a blood clot in a vein - thrombosis occurring in major veins, particularly in the extremities, is a common occurrence. Blood cannot adequately pass through the vein containing the clot, causing the blood to back up and accumulate in the body part.

2) thickening of vessel walls - as a result of various diseases, vascular walls may become swollen and thickened, which in turn lessens the size of the lumen (internal opening) of a vessel, and affects the amount of blood which can pass through.

3) pressure from an outside lesion - an external lesion, such as a tumor growing in the surrounding tissues, may press on a vein from the outside, and result in a partial or even total closure of the vascular lumen.

When localized passive hyperemia occurs, the area is generally bluish-red, swollen, and colder than normal.

Generalized passive hyperemia is normally a result of a heart disorder which affects the efficiency of the heart's pumping action. If the heart is unable to provide adequate pressure on the vascular system, blood flow has a tendency to slow down and congest up in the veins. This faulty circulation can result in blood settling to the dependent parts of the body when gravity overcomes the normal flow of blood through the circulatory system. This condition is referred to as **hypostatic congestion**. Just as post-mortem hypostasis occurs after death, and results in livor mortis, or a purplish discoloration of the tissues as a result of the pooling of the blood, hypostatic congestion can occur in the living body if circulation is sufficiently decreased. In an effort to help alleviate this condition, good medical and nursing practice dictates the frequent turning, moving, and even massaging, of bedridden patients.

When generalized passive hyperemia occurs in the systemic system, flow of blood through the pulmonary system is also diminished. When this occurs, blood is not properly oxygenated, and a resulting bluish discoloration of the tissues, known as **cyanosis,** may develop. The most common areas for cyanosis to be observed are the lips and nail beds, although more pronounced cases can show significant discoloration of the skin in general.

Thrombosis

Thrombosis is a term which refers to the formation of a solid mass, or blood clot, within the heart or vessels of the body. The mass itself is called a **thrombus.** The blood which travels through the vessels of the human body is an amazingly efficient substance, and under normal conditions is able to smoothly flow through its designated corridors while performing its vital functions. However, when various circumstances occur which adversely affect this normal flow of blood through the vessels, the blood has a tendency to clot. The most common reasons for the formation of thrombi are as follows:

1) injury to the lining of the heart or vessels - the inner lining of vessels is normally a very smooth, slick lining of epithelial tissue, and rough spots on this smooth lining often give rise to the formation of clots.

2) diseases of the blood itself - healthy blood in its normal state only forms clots when it needs to, in order to prevent abnormal loss of blood from the vascular system. Blood which is diseased, or shows some alteration in its normal composition, is predisposed to abnormal clot formation.

3) slowing of the blood flow - blood does not normally remain stagnant for any length of time, as it is always on the move in the performance of its normal functions. Slowing of the blood is another occurrence which predisposes to clotting.

When one of the above factors occurs, resulting in the formation of a thrombus, the results may be short-lived, long term, major or minor. The most common places for clots to occur are in the heart and veins of the body, but they may also develop on the arterial side of the circulatory system. (See Fig. 3). When they occur in arteries, the coronary arteries are one of the most common locations. As you can imagine, the results of thrombosis depend on where the clot is located, and to what degree a vessel is blocked. A thrombus which is attached to the vessel wall and only partially occludes the lumen is called a parietal thrombus, and one which completely blocks the vessel is referred to as an obstructive thrombus.

When arterial thrombosis occurs, it stands to reason that a decrease in blood flow to a body area may result, which is a condition known as ischemia. But, if the thrombus is located in a vein, the return of blood from a body part is affected, possibly resulting in passive hyperemia and even gangrene.

The ultimate fate of a thrombus varies a lot from case to case. It may become infected, in which case it can be called a septic thrombus, or it may be changed into a mass of fibrous tissue. Sometimes new vascular tissue develops in the thrombus to form passageways for blood to pass through, and this is called canalization. Nature's preferred way of dealing with clots is to dissolve them by means of specialized enzymes normally present in the blood. When the body is able to accomplish this, it is referred to as digestion of the thrombus. And finally, one of the worst things that can happen is for the thrombus to break loose, or break into smaller fragments, and float elsewhere in the body to create other blockages. These blockages may prove to be even more serious than the original stationary clot, and in fact often lead to such conditions as sudden strokes or heart attacks.

Embolism

Embolism refers to the condition of an object having floated through the bloodstream and causing an obstruction of a vessel. The object itself is referred to as an **embolus.** One of the most common forms of embolism occurs when a thrombus, or a piece of a thrombus, breaks loose and lodges elsewhere in the body. (See Fig. 4) Besides thrombi which become emboli, other substances may cause embolism and lead to blockages of vessels, such as the following:

1) clumps of bacteria, parasites or tumor cells - this is how infections may spread from one part of the body to another, or how a person with skin cancer may end up having brain cancer. Bacteria and tumor cells act as emboli and spread through the blood and lymph vessels.

2) fat globules - crushing injuries often result in fat globules from the tissues of the body, including yellow bone marrow, entering damaged vessels and traveling as emboli.

11

3) foreign particles - substances such as dirt, or even beebies from a shot-gun blast, can enter vessels and become emboli.

4) air or gas bubbles - bubbles may enter the circulation during operations, traumatic injuries to the chest, or through hypodermic injection.

Besides the spread of infection or tumors, the real danger of emboli is similar to that of thrombi - the blockage of vessels with a resulting decreased blood flow to a body part, which in turn may lead to death of deprived tissues. If these tissues are those of a vital organ, such as the brain or the heart muscle, the results of embolism may be sudden, serious, and even fatal. If the loss of blood supply occurs in a less vital part of the body, such as in the extremities, the result may be a slower destruction of tissue, which may in turn develop into a serious problem if left unresolved.

Ischemia and Infarction

Closely associated with the concepts of thrombosis and embolism is the term **ischemia.** Ischemia, which comes from the Greek word meaning "to hold back", refers to decreased blood flow to a body part. As we have already mentioned above, this is what often happens when a thrombus or an embolus lodges in an artery. However, ischemia may also result from other diseases, such as atherosclerosis, which causes a thickening of vascular walls, and a resulting narrowing of the arterial lumen. In addition, ischemia may result from pressure on an artery from the outside, such as when a growing tumor presses on an artery, partially or completely closing it off. Whether it results from an embolus, a thrombus, or any other cause, the overall effect of ischemia depends a lot on where it occurs, and whether or not that particular area is able to get an alternate blood supply through collateral circulation. Many areas of the body possess numerous, communicating arteries (anasto-moses), which are able to supply blood to an area which has experienced a blockage in its normal arterial channel. Therefore, areas with poor collateral circulation are more likely to suffer bad results when ischemia occurs.

When, as a result of ischemia, the area of tissue which was deprived of its blood supply dies, this is referred to as **infarc-tion.** The area of tissue which dies is called an **infarct.** Infarction may also

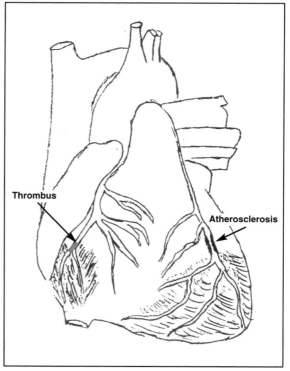

Thrombosis in coronary artery resulting in infarction (left shaded area). Atherosclerosis partially blocking coronary artery, resulting in ischemia (right shaded area).

12

be referred to as **ischemic necrosis.** When various cells of the body are subjected to a loss of oxygen as a result of their blood supply being cut off, they will eventually die. *(See Fig. 5)* Infarcts resulting from blockage of small vessels may simply be observed as a correspondingly small area of necrotic tissue, but those resulting from occlusion of a major vessel, such as a pulmonary or coronary artery, can be very serious and even fatal. Many pathologists can attest to the fact that hearts they have removed during autopsy have shown one or more infarcts, some of which may have occurred years prior to death, and only now can be observed as previously undetected areas of scarred tissue. A person may have experienced one or more minor heart attacks over the years, which did not prove fatal, but still affected the heart and its ability to perform in its most efficient manner.

Another manner in which infarction may occur is when external pressure is exerted on the surface of the body over an extended period of time, effectively cutting off the blood supply to the area being compressed. Good examples of this type of necrosis often occur on the skin and underlying tissues of bedridden patients who lie in one position for too long, and experience the common bed sores, or decubitus ulcers, on their hips, tailbones, and heels as a result. The pressure of the weight of the body continually being exerted on the underlying bedding can cause infarction to occur, and in turn the ulcerated area can become invaded by bacteria, resulting in putrefaction of the tissues. From a nursing standpoint, frequent turning and massaging of patients, plus proper padding underneath the body, can help alleviate the occurrence of bed sores, as this allows for better circulation to affected areas. From an embalmer's viewpoint, decubitus ulcers require additional care in addition to routine arterial injection. Such areas should always receive supplemental treatment in the form of cavity packs, and/or direct hypodermic injection of disinfectant and preservative chemicals into the affected area, followed by the use of drying agents and bandaging as necessary.

Gangrene

Gangrene is often classified as either dry gangrene or moist (true) gangrene. **Dry gangrene** is not a preferred term, as it is not really gangrene at all, but simply another name for ischemic necrosis. The term is most often used when ischemic necrosis occurs in the extremities, particularly the foot and lower leg area. The affected part is dry, shrunken, and progressively turns darker in color until it is completely black. If an area of dry gangrene is invaded by saprophytic bacteria, it may turn into moist gangrene.

Moist or **true gangrene** is characterized by necrotic tissue which has been invaded by bacteria, which in turn are responsible for the putrefaction that occurs. As the name implies, moist gangrene is characterized by a swollen, high liquid content of the tissues, with bad odors and a tendency to spread. Severe cases of moist gangrene often require amputation of part of an extremity in order to prevent the entire limb from being lost, or even causing death.

Besides occurring as a progression of dry gangrene, moist gangrene is often associated with disturbances in the venous return of blood from an area. Diseases or injuries which damage the vascular system in a given area, and result in blood stagnation and improper drainage from the vicinity, may predispose to moist gangrene. Examples of such conditions include crushing injuries of the toes and feet, or freezing of the tissues which occurs during frostbite. Also, diabetes mellitus is a disease which is often complicated by damage to the vascular walls, with resulting poor circulation, and a predispo-

13

sition for gangrene occurring, particularly in the extremities, where circulation is the most likely to be sluggish. *(See Fig. 6)*

Hemorrhage

Hemorrhage is defined as the escape of blood from the vascular system. Any time that blood leaves a vessel, it can be described as hemorrhage. The main reason that blood would escape from a blood vessel is due to a break in the walls of the vessel. When a vascular wall is traumatized, such as from cutting by a sharp object, or rupturing as a result of blunt force, blood is likely to escape into the surrounding tissue or onto a body surface. This type of bleeding is sometimes called hemorrhage per rhexis, from the Greek word for "rupture". However, blood occasionally escapes through vascular walls which are not obviously broken, but as a result of a weakening or a disease of the vessel walls, blood is able to seep out. In addition to diseased vascular walls, blood could possibly escape from the vessels due to some disease of the blood itself. When the escape of blood occurs in one of these situations, and the vascular walls are not actually broken, it can be referred to as hemorrhage per diapedesis. Remember, white blood cells are supposed to be able to perform diapedesis in order to attack bacteria invading the tissues of the body, but when red blood cells escape from vessels via diapedesis, this qualifies as hemorrhage.

Hemorrhages are often identified based on their appearance, such as when they occur as tiny, "pin-point" hemorrhages, and are referred to as **petechiae** (Italian meaning flea bite). The term **ecchymosis** is given to larger irregular patches of hemorrhage in the tissues, and is sometimes referred to as a bruise when occurring under the skin. **Purpura,** from the Latin word "purple", describes widespread areas of hemorrhage into the skin or mucous membranes. A **hematoma** is a tumor-like swelling filled with blood. *(See Fig. 7).* An example of a hematoma is the common blood blister. **Melena,** from the Greek word for "black", refers to very dark, tarry feces or vomitus, which results from the action of gastro-intestinal secretions upon blood in the digestive tract.

Hemorrhages are also identified based on where they occur, such as the following examples:

1) **Hemothorax** - bleeding into the pleural cavity

2) **Hemopericardium** - bleeding into the pericardial cavity–*(See Fig. 8)*

3) **Hemoperitoneum** - bleeding into the peritoneal cavity

4) **Hemoptysis** - blood in the sputum(or from the lungs)

5) **Hematemesis** - blood in the vomit (or from the stomach)

6) **Epistaxis** - bleeding from the nose

When normal, healthy blood is contained within the vascular system, it flows easily through the vessels and remains in its fluid form. However, when hemorrhage occurs, the blood is fairly rapidly converted into a soft, jelly-like mass known as a clot. The physiological process of blood clotting is essential to life, keeping us from losing excess amounts of blood when injury to the vessels occurs. This process of blood changing from a liquid, free flowing form, into a semi-solid state is called **coagulation.**

The coagulation of blood is a complicated chemical process, involving a series of events which eventually results in the closing of the break in the vessel wall by the clot which is formed. The clotting process begins when blood platelets congregate at the site of damage, and platelet factors are released. In addition, damaged tissue cells release substances called thromboplastin. Platelet factors and thromboplastin, in concert with calcium present in the blood, acts upon the blood protein prothrombin, changing it into thrombin. In turn, thrombin acts upon the blood protein fibrinogen to form fibrin, which is a meshwork of strands, or fibers, and serves to snare red blood cells and form the clot. Although this coagulation synopsis represents the basic process of clotting, scientists have identified at least thirteen separate factors or events which occur during the blood clotting process.

Circulatory Shock

Shock is a term used to describe the condition which results from a serious reduction of blood flow in the body, resulting in reduced oxygen supply to the tissues. It is often described as a state of collapse with depressed vital signs. A person with shock often displays a weak, rapid pulse, low blood pressure, shallow breathing, and cold and clammy skin, especially in the extremities. Many circumstances may lead to shock, and there are several subcategories of the condition, such as cardiogenic shock, where the heart fails to pump blood through the circulatory system, or hemorrhagic shock, due to a loss of blood supply in the body. Other conditions, such as serious infection, poisoning, and dehydration can also lead to shock.

Fainting, or syncope, has often been described as a mild form of shock, due to a temporary decrease of blood flow to the brain. It may be interpreted as a nervous reaction affecting the vascular system, and may be elicited by such things as pain or emotion, even minor in nature. For instance, fainting often accompanies such occurrences as the sight of blood, fear of hypodermic injections, or strong grief situations.

Edema and Fluid Balance

A recollection of basic anatomy reminds us that much of the fluid in the human body is not static, but constantly on the move and changing positions. When blood plasma seeps out of capillary walls to bathe the tissues of the body, it is referred to as tissue fluid. When this tissue fluid moves into tiny lymph vessels, eventually to be returned to the bloodstream, it is referred to as lymph. During a state of health, the amount and location of these basic body fluids remains fairly constant. However, various disease conditions can significantly alter this normal balance of body fluids, and result in chemical changes of these fluids, or simply changes in where various amounts of fluid are located at a given time.

The condition called **edema** refers to an excess accumulation of fluid in the tissues of the body. Edema is an extravascular condition, where tissue fluid is not progressing out of the intercellular spaces of the body and back into the lymph vessels or capillaries. Tissues may become so waterlogged in edema that they take on a "doughy" consistency, and retain the impression of a fingerprint when pressed upon, in which case it may be referred to as "pitting" edema.

Edema may be either localized in a limited anatomical area of the body, or widespread throughout the tissues. Several of the main causes of edema are as follows:

1) heart failure

2) venous or lymphatic obstruction

3) increased capillary permeability, such as that which occurs during inflammations

4) decreased osmotic pressure of plasma proteins

When the main pump forcing blood through the circulatory system, the heart, fails to function properly, blood has a tendency to slow down and back up in the venous side of the circulatory system. If you recall, this was described earlier as generalized passive hyperemia. When this happens, blood plasma which has seeped out into the tissues is not allowed back into the capillaries due to the excess amount of blood already there. Therefore, it tends to remain in the intercellular spaces, causing generalized edema. From the Greek words meaning throughout (ana-) and flesh (sarco-), we get the term **anasarca,** which is the name given to generalized or widespread edema.

Also discussed earlier in the chapter was the concept of localized passive hyperemia occurring in a body part as a result of blockage of a vein. When this happens, or when a major lymph duct is blocked, impairing the drainage of tissue fluid through the lymphatic system, localized edema may result. For instance, if blood is backing up in the right leg because a thrombus is occluding the femoral vein, it is likely that edema will develop in the area as a result. If the fluid build-up in the tissues is from a lymphatic duct being obstructed, it could be referred to as lymphedema.

A capillary wall normally has what is called "selective permeability", meaning that some substances such as fluids easily pass through, but larger protein molecules are retained in the bloodstream. During inflammations, capillaries lose some of this selective permeability and greater amounts of these blood proteins, and additional fluids, pass into the tissues and accumulate, resulting in localized edema. The term **exudate** is given to edema which collects around an inflammation site.

Certain blood proteins, especially serum albumin, are responsible for maintaining the proper osmotic pressure between the blood and the surrounding fluid in the tissues. If blood albumin levels fall below a certain point, the osmotic pressure of the blood decreases, causing the water in the blood to pass out of the vessels and into the surrounding tissues, where the osmotic pressure is higher. Consequently, edema occurs in the tissues as a result of this imbalance in osmotic pressures. Albumin can be lost from the bloodstream for several reasons, including kidney inflammation which results in the loss of excess amounts of albumin through the urinary system, or the inability of the liver to properly produce albumin for one reason or another.

Like hemorrhages, many edemas are named based on their location, such as **hydrothorax,** meaning edema of the pleural cavity, **hydropericardium,** meaning edema of the pericardial cavity, or **ascites,** which refers to edema of the peritoneal cavity. Ascites comes from the Greek word for "sack or bag", and in this case the sack being referred to is the peritoneum, which surrounds and anchors most of the abdominal organs.

The various anatomic areas of the healthy human body contain a fairly normal and constant amount of fluids, particularly water. Water makes up approximately seventy percent of all body fluids and is present as intravascular fluid within the vessels, extravascular fluid outside of the vessels and between the individual cells of the body, and is also present as intracellular fluid within the cells. The proper balance of water in these anatomic areas is important to homeostasis of the body's internal environment and is a function of both water intake and output. If water intake is too low, or output too high, **dehydration** can occur. Dehydration, also known as **desiccation,** can be defined as a decrease in total body fluids, and can be a serious and even fatal condition if it progresses beyond certain levels. Failure to take in adequate amounts of water is fairly easy to understand, whereas some of the reasons for loss of excess fluids are somewhat more complicated. Additionally, proper levels of salt in the body are important, as salt has a direct impact on the retention of water in bodily tissues. Loss of large amounts of salt can aggravate the problem of dehydration by causing additional water to be lost from the body. Some of the more common reasons for dehydration are as follows:

1) high body temperature during febrile diseases, which leads to moisture loss via sweating through the skin

2) high environmental temperatures, which also cause excessive sweating

3) gastro-intestinal diseases which result in either considerable vomiting or diarrhea

4) glandular diseases which exhibit hormonal disturbances. Various hormones have regulatory effects on water and salt levels in the body, such as the anti-diuretic hormone secreted by the posterior part of the pituitary gland, which regulates the amount of water lost through the urinary system. Also, decreased levels of aldosterone, an adrenal cortex hormone, can lead to loss of excessive amounts of salt through the urinary system, which in turn causes dehydration

Science has learned over the years that replenishment of water without a corresponding replenishment of salts can upset the normal osmotic concentration of the fluid in the tissues of the body. A good example of this happening is the cramping of muscles which often occurs in athletes who have lost a lot of water and salt through sweating. Drinking of extra fluids, plus intake of additional salt, can help prevent or alleviate these so called "heat cramps". As a result of this knowledge, it can be observed that many athletes now attempt to replenish bodily fluids through the use of various commercially available sports drinks, which include essential salts and other substances besides just water.

Embalming Implications Associated With Circulatory Disorders

From the perspective of an embalmer, circulatory disorders can pose some of the most important concerns which may affect the successful outcome of the embalming operation.

Diminished circulation to an area is a prime concern for the embalmer. Diseases of the circulatory system, such as thrombosis, embolism, tumors, and various other arterial disorders to be discussed later, can result in the flow of embalming fluids to the body parts being significantly decreased. Such occurrences will require that the embalmer use the proper fluids and techniques in order to improve distribution to all body areas. Diminished circulation may even have the effect of causing **dehydration and emaciation** of various body areas if the blood supply has been lessened for an extended period of time.

Hemorrhage may also occur as a result of circulatory disorders, effectively short-circuiting the flow of embalming fluid through the body. This in turn may lead to **swelling** and blood **discolorations,** which can further complicate the process of embalming. These conditions may be lessened by the use of such techniques as multiple injection sites, dehydrating or bleaching fluids, proper massage techniques, and the use of external cosmetics.

When circulatory conditions such as passive hyperemia and **edema** exist, they require the embalming operator to closely consider the type and quantity of arterial solution to be used. Edematous bodies have the effect of causing increased secondary dilution of embalming solutions, and this must be taken into consideration when selecting the proper fluids to be used. In addition, edematous fluid in the tissues predisposes to more **rapid decomposition** in a dead body. Gangrene may even be present in some bodies which experience serious circulatory disorders, as is often the case with chronic and severe diabetes mellitus. Gangrene in turn presents the embalmer with an extra problem of treating an area of discoloration, putrefaction, and bad odors.

Abscesses are also often associated with the destruction and degeneration of tissues as a result of circulatory interruption. Whenever possible, abscesses should receive special care, such as aspiration of pus prior to embalming, and subsequent treatment to ensure proper disinfection and preservation of tissues in the area of the abscess.

Chapter Three
Regressive Tissue Changes

Regressive tissue changes may be described as the various pathological processes indicating some disturbance in cell metabolism. If the normal metabolic activities of a cell are disturbed, it is likely that altered function and structure may result, with necrosis, or death of the cell, being the ultimate outcome if the process is not arrested in time. Some of the main regressive tissue changes affecting the body are infiltrations, degenerations, and atrophy.

As the name implies, **infiltration** suggests that some sort of substance has infiltrated the tissues of the body and accumulated in abnormal amounts. One of the more common forms of infiltration occurs when coloring matters pass into the tissues and accumulate, causing discolorations. This is referred to as **pigmentation.** Pigmentations are further categorized based on whether the coloring matter is from a normal pigment present in the body, in which case it would be called an **endogenous** (Latin endo meaning inside), or from a pigment which entered the body from outside, in which case it would be called an **exogenous** pigmentation (Latin exo meaning outside).

Pigmentations

Endogenous	Exogenous
Bilirubin - Jaundice	Coal dust - Anthracosis
Melanin - Melanosis	Stone dust - Silicosis
Hemoglobin - Blood discolorations	Cotton dust - Byssinosis

Endogenous pigments include **bilirubin,** which is an orange to yellowish pigment present in bile. Bile is a digestive juice produced by the liver, and is involved in emulsifying fats in the digestive tract. Various diseases, such as liver cancer, inflammations, and blockages of the bile ducts, can result in this bile pigment spilling over into the bloodstream. When this occurs, bilirubin collects in the tissues, causing a yellowish discoloration of the skin, the whites of the eyes, and other areas. This characteristic yellow discoloration is referred to as **jaundice** or **icterus.**

Hemoglobin is another endogenous pigment, normally functioning as the oxygen carrying substance within a red blood cell. A good example of pigmentation caused by hemoglobin is post-mortem stain, which results from the post-mortem hemolysis of red blood cells. This hemolysis, in turn, results in the liberation of hemoglobin from the red cells, and eventually a staining, or pigmentation, of the tissues can occur.

A third form of endogenous pigmentation can occur when abnormal amounts of **melanin,** the normal brownish coloring matter present in the skin, accumulates in the tissues. Melanosis is a term given to unusual deposits of patches of melanin in different parts of the body. Even the common freckle and mole are examples of excess melanin being present in certain areas of the skin.

Exogenous pigmentations, or those originating outside of the body, can probably be best demonstrated by considering the various dusts which infiltrate the lungs and accumulate to cause discolorations. These pigmentations caused by prolonged inhalation of dust are referred to as **pneumoconiosis.** Examples of pneumoconiosis are those caused by coal dust (**anthracosis**) and stone dust (**silicosis**). Anthracosis, commonly called black lung disease, is associated with the occupation of coal mining. Silicosis, from the word "silicon", is associated with other types of jobs involving such activities as sandblasting or quarrying of various minerals. Those who live in areas where textile mills are important industries may be familiar with a condition called "mill fever" or "brown lung" disease, resulting from inhalation of cotton dust and related foreign materials over the years. This condition is scientifically referred to as **byssinosis,** from the Greek word for cotton.

Degeneration is a general term referring to the deterioration of cells within the body due to changes which occur within the cytoplasm of the cells, and which affects their normal function. For one reason or another, normal cellular metabolism is impaired, or is unable to manage the accumulation of various substances within the cell. For example, one common form of degeneration is called **fatty degeneration**, because fatty molecules are accumulating within cells and having an adverse effect on normal cellular function. The liver is an example of an organ often affected by fatty degeneration, as it is directly involved with normal fat metabolism in the body. A liver affected by this condition may be enlarged, yellowish in color, and greasy to the touch. (*See Fig. 9*)

Another form of degeneration is **amyloid disease**, or amyloidosis, where a waxy, starch-like substance called amyloid is deposited in the tissues. It is thought to be a metabolic disorder involving proteins, and may accompany various chronic, pathological conditions.

Cloudy swelling (cellular swelling) is a term often given to the appearance cells take on when they are somewhat swollen and contain an abnormal amount of water. It is a fairly common degenerative condition, often accompanying even minor illnesses and injuries, and is not usually as serious as other forms of degeneration.

Pathological **calcification** is a condition in which calcium is deposited within the tissues of the body with no attempt at bone formation. Calcium is normally deposited in bone, but when it infiltrates other tissues, particularly those which are already dead or dying, or are degenerative in some form, it is referred to as pathological calcification. Good examples of calcification occurring are when calcium is deposited in the vascular walls during arteriosclerosis, and when the lesions of tuberculosis, called tubercles, become hardened with calcium.

Atrophy is a term which refers to the decrease in size of a once normal body part. It should not be confused with hypoplasia, which indicates underdevelopment of a body part. In hypoplasia, the body part never properly developed in the first place. Atrophy may be either physiological or pathological in nature. Physiological atrophy, which indicates that the decrease in size is a normal, regular occurrence in the human body, can be seen in such examples as atrophy of the mammary glands after milk production ceases, atrophy of the uterus after pregnancy, or general atrophy with old age, sometimes referred to as senile atrophy. In addition, the thymus gland, which is a mass of lymphoid tissue located behind the upper portion of the sternum, and is important in the early development of the immune system in a child, characteristically atrophies after puberty, and becomes a shriveled, functionless mass of tissue in the adult.

Pathological atrophy may occur as a result of various functional and structural problems which occur in the different organs of the body. Some of the more common reasons which give rise to pathological atrophy are as follows:

1) inadequate nutrition - this can be observed as a generalized condition in cases such as starvation, or a localized condition when blood supply is decreased to a body part. Without the proper nutrients the bloodstream

delivers to the various bodily parts, maintenance of the normal structure, function, and size of tissues may be impaired. (*See Fig. 10*)

2) inadequate nervous stimulation - if normal nervous control over certain muscle groups, for example, is interrupted, atrophy may occur. Muscles require nervous stimulation in order to contract and create movement, thus performing their normal function. This can be seen in many disease conditions which result in paralysis of body parts and consequently a decrease in size of the area due to the loss of function.

3) disuse - a good example of atrophy from disuse can be seen when a broken arm or leg spends 8 - 10 weeks in a cast, disallowing normal use of the limb during that period of time. After removal of the cast, it can usually be seen that the affected area emerges from this period of disuse considerably smaller and weaker than its healthy counterpart.

Chapter Four

Inflammation

Inflammation may be defined as the body's response to tissue injury. Whenever a sufficient quantity of living cells are damaged, a rather complex series of physiological events is triggered in the body, in an attempt to correct the adverse condition which exists. Inflammation itself is not a disease, but a process the body goes through in responding to the fact that injury has occurred. Inflammation may be thought of as a defense mechanism, whose purpose is threefold: To destroy and remove the injurious agent from the body; to limit the extension of this injurious agent in the body; and to serve as the mechanism for allowing the body to repair itself and return the injured tissues to normal use.

Certainly many things can serve as agents for injury to the tissues of the body. Some of the more common causes of inflammation are as follows:

1) living agents - microorganisms such as bacteria, fungi, protozoa, and viruses are often a major cause of injury to the tissues. When inflammation is caused by living agents, it is generally referred to as **infection.**

2) chemical irritants - chemicals such as strong acids or alkalis are capable of causing significant damage to bodily tissues.

3) physical irritants - this general category of tissue injury includes a variety of agents, such as heat and cold, electricity, radiation injuries, and trauma. Trauma involves physical injuries such as fractures, bruises, cuts, and gunshots.

4) immunological reactions - inflammation may be caused by the action of antibodies which a person has produced acting upon their own tissues. Sometimes the body's immune system can fail to distinguish between what is natural tissue and what is a foreign antigen, and a reaction can occur causing damage to various tissues. These conditions are often referred to as autoimmune diseases.

Regardless which of these basic causative agents is involved, the common underlying situation is damage to bodily tissues. The inflammation process is generally initiated when injured and dying cells release chemical substances into the surrounding tissues which in turn stimulate other events to occur. Part of what occurs may be described as a **vascular** response, in that tiny blood vessels in the area dilate, and increased blood flow is allowed into the vicinity. This may be interpreted as **active pathological hyperemia** occurring as a result of the inflammation process. As the capillaries at the site become more permeable, they leak additional fluid into the area, which carries with it various substances such as antibodies, and plasma proteins which will be involved in the formation of fibrin, in an attempt to form a barrier against the spread of the injurious agent. These fluids which collect around an inflammation site may be thought of as a type of edema, and are referred to as **exudates.** Exudates are often subcategorized based on the substances they contain. They may be called purulent or suppurative if they contain pus, hemorrhagic if they contain blood or serous if they contain only the clear liquid portion of the blood.

In addition to the vascular response which occurs, a **cellular** response is also involved in the inflammation process. Via the process of **diapedesis,** white blood cells are migrating out of the capillary walls and into the surrounding tissues. These cells, particularly neutrophils, are involved in **phagocytosis,** and help to ingest invading bacteria and other cellular debris. The phagocytic activity of the body's white cells is critical to clearing the way for the eventual repair of the damaged tissues, and hopefully their return to normal use.

In many forms of inflammation, certain bacteria cause the formation of **pus,** which results from the liquefaction of dead tissue cells, and the action of white blood cells attempting to fight off the invading bacteria. Thus, pus can be presumed to contain both fluid and a mixture of living and dead tissue, plus bacterial and white blood cells. The process of pus formation is called **suppuration.** Bacteria which cause suppuration are referred to as **pyogenic** (pyo = pus, gen = producing) bacteria. Some of the more common pyogenic bacteria include *Staphylococcus aureus, Streptococcus pyogenes, Pseudomonas aeruginosa,* and *Neisseria gonorrhea.*

Inflammation has several important signs associated with it, which are usually referred to as the "cardinal signs of inflammation". They include **heat** (calor), **redness** (rubor), **pain** (dolor), **swelling** (tumor), and **altered function.** Heat and redness are associated with the extra blood flow normally present at the inflammation site, and swelling results from the additional blood flow as well as the presence of exudates in the area. Pain can be attributed to pressure on, and irritation of, sensory nerve endings in the vicinity. And, of course, altered function, or even loss of function, can result from any combination of these factors interfering with the normal physiology of the body parts involved.

Following is a list of some of the more common lesions associated with inflammation:

1) **abscess** - an area of pus surrounded by a wall of inflammatory tissue *(See Fig. 11)*

2) **ulcer** - a localized area of necrosis on the skin or mucous membrane *(See Fig. 12)*

3) **vesicle** - an elevation on the skin containing fluid, as in a blister

4) **pustule** - an elevation on the skin containing pus, as in a pimple

5) **furuncle** or boil - an abscess located in the deeper layers of the skin

6) **carbuncle** - two or more communicating furuncles, and often accompanied by additional symptoms such as fever, leukocytosis, weakness, and fatigue

When the inflammation process (possibly with the aid of modern antibiotics) has managed to overcome the injurious agent in the body, the next step is to set about repairing damaged tissue, and returning the body part to its original state if possible. Although this process is a rather complex and orderly one, it can be presumed that either the area of damaged tissue is returned precisely to its former state, or it is not, and some different arrangement of tissues has replaced the original one. A lot of what happens during this healing process depends on how severe the damage was to the original tissue. The term **repair** is often used to describe the replacement of damaged tissue with connective tissue. For example, if a wound is minor, or its edges can be readily drawn together in order to promote the healing process, little or no scarring may occur. However, more serious wounds may result in the body's use of fibrous connective tissue to fill in the gaps resulting in the formation of a scar or **cicatrix.** Scars contain no blood vessels, hair follicles, oil or sweat glands, or nerve endings.

Regeneration, on the other hand, refers to the replacement of damaged tissue with identical tissue. Some tissues in the body have greater regenerative capacity than others, so whether or not regeneration can occur depends not only on the severity of the tissue damage that occurs, but also on the type of tissue which was destroyed. As a general rule, connective and epithelial tissues regenerate fairly well, muscles regenerate poorly, and nervous tissue the least well of all. If the nerve cell bodies are destroyed, they will never regenerate, but their processes may regenerate over time if the cell body was not severely damaged. The term resolution is used to indicate the termination of an inflammatory reaction, with the body part returned to normal use.

We can all relate to this repair and regeneration process, as each of us can likely point to this scar or that one which highlights some past traumatic injury we received. But we can also point to natural, normal looking skin, which has, at one time or another, been nicked, scraped, burned, or otherwise injured, only to regenerate itself and return to its former state with no adverse, long-term effects. If this were not the case, we would each end up walking masses of scar tissue by the time we reach old age!

Inflammation and Repair Process

Causative Agent

(e.g. Bacteria)

Cellular Damage Occurs

Chemicals Released from Dying Cells

Bodily Responses Occur

-Active Pathological Hyperemia

-Leukocytosis/Phagocytosis

-Exudates form

-Fever and antibody production increased

-Suppuration may occur

Containment and Neutralization

of Causative Agent Occurs

Regeneration

of

Damaged Cells

Repair/Fibrosis/Cicatrix

Formation

Resolution

Resolution

Embalming Implications of Inflammation

The presence of any form of inflammation in or on a dead human body should alert the embalmer to the fact that careful attention, and often additional care, is needed to treat the situation. As we have previously noted, inflammation can affect any area of the body, and the after effects of various inflammations can present the embalmer with special concerns. For example, surface conditions such as skin burns, either from heat or chemicals, must generally receive special treatment, ranging from cosmetic covering of minor discolorations, to more extensive treatment of badly damaged tissues, including excision of necrotic tissue, surface compresses and hypodermic injection to supplement arterial injection, and deep wound filling and waxing when necessary. Infectious lesions such as abscesses and ulcerations should be similarly treated in order to assure adequate disinfection and preservation of the tissues involved. Likewise, any time there is an indication of an internal inflammatory condition, the respective area, whether it's the mouth and throat area, the lungs, the digestive tract, or any other anatomical location, should receive special attention by the embalmer. The embalmer should proceed under the assumption that any body which was afflicted with inflammation in any form is likely to be a reservoir of increased bacterial activity, higher fluid content in localized areas of inflammation, and generally in need of treatment above and beyond routine arterial injection and drainage.

Chapter Five

Neoplasms

From the Greek words "neo" meaning new and "plasm", referring to a formed substance, we get the term **neoplasm.** A neoplasm is any new, abnoral growth of tissue in the body which serves no useful purpose. Normal tissue growth in the human body is an orderly, controlled process, which occurs on a predictable basis, and within certain established guidelines. Neoplasms do not fall within this general category of growth, but seem to grow and result in cellular proliferation completely separate from other normal body tissues. The term **tumor** literally means a swelling, and although all tumors are not necessarily neoplasms, the terms tumor and neoplasm have come to be used somewhat interchangeably. The study of neoplasms or tumors is referred to as **oncology.**

There are several other terms which are often used when describing growth of bodily tissues, but are not considered neoplastic in nature. One of these terms is **hypertrophy,** which is used to describe an increase in the size of a body part due to an increase in the size of the individual cells. For example, exercise and weight training will increase the size of the body's muscles by increasing the size of individual muscle fibers, not the number of muscle cells present in the body. It can be said that increased functional demand on an organ may result in hypertrophy of that organ. Occasionally, when an organ increases in size due to the failure of another organ (or part of an organ), it is referred to as compensatory hypertrophy. For example, a kidney or lung may hypertrophy to some degree after the loss of its "partner" in order to compensate for the extra workload which is being demanded of it.

Unlike hypertrophy, **hyperplasia** refers to an increase in the size of a body part due to an increase in the number of cells in that organ. This type of size increase often occurs in endocrine glands which produce hormones necessary to regulate various bodily functions. If additional thyroid hormone is needed in the body, the gland may undergo hyperplasia to the degree necessary to meet this demand. However, unlike neoplasia, this type of increased growth is of a limited, controlled nature.

One other form of tissue growth to be mentioned is metaplasia, which refers to a replacement of one type of tissue in a major category (e.g., epithelial) by another type of tissue in that same category. In other words, one type of epithelial tissue, such as squamous cells, may replace another type of epithelium, such as columnar cells. This is often seen in the lining of the respiratory passageways after chronic inflammations or long term smoking. These irritations result in the loss of the normal type of epithelium found in this location with another type not normally found there. In addition, this second type of tissue may not be equally suited to perform the physiological functions intended at this location, which may in turn lead to functional disturbances and problems in the future.

Classification of Tumors

Tumors are often discussed and categorized based on two major areas: A clinical basis, meaning how they behave and their general characteristics, and a histological basis, meaning the type of tissue from which the tumors arise.

Considering first the clinical basis for classifying tumors, there are two major subcategories of tumors, which are called **malignant** and **benign.** Benign tumors, from the Latin word for "mild", are the less serious ones, and malignant tumors, from the Latin meaning "of bad kind", are the more serious, life threatening type–those we would normally refer to as cancers. The term **cancer** is used to refer to any malignant neoplasm.

Benign and malignant tumors differ from each other in a number of significant ways. Following is a list of some of the more important distinctions:

1) Benign tumors are said to grow by **expansion.** They expand as they grow and push aside surrounding tissues, but do not infiltrate or invade these tissues. Malignant tumors, on the other hand, grow by **infiltration.** They do not just expand from the center outward as do benign tumors, but they grow from the edges, and send out processes or strands like the claws of a crab which dig into the surrounding tissues. The word cancer comes from the Latin word for "crab", due to the appearance of a malignant tumor with its crab-like extensions which infiltrate other tissues.

2) As a result of their expansive type of growth, benign tumors are often **encapsulated.** This capsule represents a reactive process on the part of the body as a result of the pressure exerted on surrounding tissues. Malignant tumors generally are not encapsulated and the body has greater trouble surrounding, walling off, and controlling the invasive nature of these tumors.

3) Benign tumors do not generally spread from their original growth site. Malignancies, however, are well known for their ability to spread from one body area to another. The term **metastasis** is used to describe the ability of malignant tumors to spread. By infiltrating surrounding blood and lymph capillaries, tumor cells are carried to other body locations where new tumors are formed. When cancerous cells are carried away from a site by lymph vessels, they are likely to be trapped in a regional lymph node, which may itself succumb to the malignancy and eventually be destroyed. When surgery is done to remove malignant tumors, it is often necessary to also remove surrounding lymph nodes where cancer cells are likely to be located. By doing so, the chances of these cells eventually reaching the bloodstream, and being more widely dispersed, is greatly reduced.

4) Benign tumors generally do not cause extensive destruction of tissues, whereas malignant tumors do cause great damage to surrounding tissues.

5) Although all tumor cells are altered cells, with the ability to grow more rapidly than normal cells, individual cells in a benign tumor usually bear a fairly close resemblance to the tissue from which they originated. In malignant tumors, this is not the case. Cancerous cells are often greatly different microscopically from their tissue of origin. Generally speaking, the more different the cells of a tumor are from their original tissue, the more likely they are to be malignant.

6) Benign tumors generally do not recur when surgically removed. As previously mentioned, they are usually encapsulated, and the entire tumor can be excised without leaving behind unnoticed portions of the tumor. Malignant tumors often recur after surgery, due to the difficult chore of removing the main part of the tumor, plus its extensions into surrounding tissues.

7) Benign tumors are not normally fatal. However, they can be quite serious if their anatomic location results in interference with the function of a vital organ, or puts pressure on a major nerve or blood vessel serving a

particular body area. Malignant tumors are very likely to become fatal if not removed or properly treated. The success of modern medicine in treating various malignancies varies a great degree depending on the type of tumor involved. Highly successful treatment, approaching 100%, has been accomplished for some tumors, whereas poor success rates remain with others.

The second main focus in the classification of tumors is the histological basis, meaning what type of tissue the tumor originated from. In the naming of tumors, there are some general guidelines which can be observed, and which can help us identify the type of tumor by understanding the usage of certain word endings. While there are numerous exceptions to the rule, tumors whose names end simply in "oma" are usually benign. The suffix "sarcoma" is used to identify malignancies of non-epithelial tissues, especially various connective and muscle tissue tumors. The ending "carcinoma" designates malignancies of epithelial tissue. Bearing these general rules in mind, we can approach the study of various tumors based on their classification as benign or malignant, plus the type of tissue they arise from. In the following list, we will use the designation (b) to indicate benign tumors, and (m) to indicate malignant tumors.

Connective Tissue Tumors

1) Osteoma (b) and osteosarcoma (m) - tumors of bone

2) Fibroma (b) and fibrosarcoma (m) - tumors of fibrous connective tissue (*See Fig. 13*)

3) Chondroma (b) and chondrosarcoma (m) - tumors of cartilage

4) Lipoma (b) and liposarcoma (m) - tumors of fatty or adipose tissue (*See Fig. 14*)

5) Angioma (b) and angiosarcoma (m) - these are tumors of vessels, and are generally subcategorized based on the type of vessel involved. Lymphangiomas (b) and lymph-angio-sarcomas (m) are tumors of lymph vessels, whereas hemangiomas(b) and hemangiosarcomas(m) are tumors of blood vessels. The common red or purplish birthmarks often found in the skin, sometimes referred to as "port-wine stains", are examples of capillary hemangiomas.

6) Lymphoma (m) or lymphosarcoma (m) - tumors of lymphoid tissue, or lymph nodes. As most lymphoid tissue tumors are malignant, the term lymphoma is assumed to indicate a malignant tumor, even though it has only the -oma ending. **Hodgkin's disease** is a form of lymphoma usually striking young adult males. The prognosis for lymphomas has improved dramatically in recent years, assuming proper treatment is administered in the early stages of the disease.

7) Leukemia (m) - although not a tumor as such, leukemia is a malignancy of the hemopoietic (blood forming) tissues of the body, such as the bone marrow. It is sometimes referred to as "cancer of the blood". It is usually characterized by a massive and uncontrolled leukocytosis, or increase in white blood cells. Whereas a normal white cell count is 7-9,000 per cubic millimeter, in leukemia the count often reaches into the hundreds of thousands per cubic millimeter, with many of the white cells being immature and abnormal forms. A moderate and temporary, or transient leukocytosis, is normal in times of infection, and is an important defense

mechanism of the body, unlike the relatively permanent and massive leukocytosis associated with leukemia.

Epithelial Tissue Tumors

1) Adenoma (b) and adenocarcinoma (m)–tumors of glandular epithelium - this includes tumors of certain organs whose cells produce various secretions, such as the breast, prostate, and thyroid glands.

2) Epithelioma (m) or squamous cell carcinoma (m)–tumors of stratified squamous epithelium, wherever it occurs. It is fairly common in such areas as the skin, lung, mouth, and uterus.

3) Basal cell carcinoma (m)–another malignancy of epithelial tissue in the skin, differing somewhat in structure from a squamous cell carcinoma. It generally occurs on the face, and is slower growing and less malignant than a squamous cell carcinoma.

4) Transitional cell carcinoma (m)–a carcinoma affecting the form of epithelial tissue lining the urinary tract. It is common in the ureters, urethra, and urinary bladder.

5) Papilloma (b)–although they may turn malignant, papillomas are generally benign tumors of epithelial tissue in the skin and mucous membranes. Those which are covered with a hard, rough layer of stratified squamous epithelium are commonly referred to as **warts.** Warts are papillomas which are viral in origin. A **polyp** is a form of papilloma which grows with a "pedicle", or stem, from the underlying tissue. They are quite common in the stomach, intestinal tract, and nasal areas. *(See Fig. 15)*

6) Nevus (b) or melanoma (m)–a nevus is a tumor, usually congenital, which arises in the skin and contains an abundance of melanin, the normal brownish coloring matter present in the skin. Hence, they are referred to as pigmented tumors, commonly called **moles,** and they generally grow to a certain point and remain there without harm. However, they sometimes develop into a highly malignant form called a **melanoma.** Moles which increase in size, change color, or become painful and bleed, should be immediately referred to a physician for evaluation.

Tumors of Muscle

1) Myoma (b) and myosarcoma (m)–these are tumors of muscle tissue, and are usually subcategorized based on the type of muscle tissue from which they arise. Leiomyomas (b) and leiomyosarcomas (m) are those which affect smooth, or involuntary muscle, such as that in the uterus or along the alimentary canal. Rhabdomyomas (b) and rhabdomyosarcomas (m), which are much less common than those affecting smooth muscle, affect voluntary or striated muscle tissue.

Tumors of Nervous Tissue

1) Neuroma (b)–tumors involving nerve cells

2) Glioma (m)–tumors involving the neuroglia, which is the supporting tissue of the nervous system, separating the individual neurons. Primary brain tumors most often involve the neuroglia, not individual neurons, and do not metastasize but kill by invading and destroying surrounding nervous tissue.

Causes of Cancer

Although the exact cause of cancer is still unknown, there are many factors which science has been able to identify which are involved in the process of tumor formation. The term **carcinogen** is usually given to any agent capable of causing cancer. Following is a discussion of some of the factors believed to be important as carcinogenic agents.

1) Heredity - although there are many studies which have contradicted each other concerning the importance of genetics in causing cancer, scientists have shown that there are some situations which tend to support the fact that heredity does play a factor in the likelihood of certain individuals contracting cancer. Breast cancer is one example of a tumor which is more likely to occur in women whose family members have also had the disease.

2) Environmental factors - many factors in our daily environment are thought to be carcinogenic, such as exposure to dusts of various types. A prime example is the problem of asbestos particles causing lung cancer in those who have been exposed to this agent over long periods of time. Probably no more has been studied and written about carcinogenic agents than that of smoke, especially the smoke from cigarettes and other tobacco products. The foods we eat are also frequently implicated as carcinogenic agents, often as a result of processing methods, the use of food additives, or the presence of pesticides and other chemicals used in our agricultural industries. Another environmental factor which has been shown to be involved in the production of cancer cells is excessive radiation. A good example of this is seen with long-term exposure to ultra-violet rays from the sun, which scientists believe is an important factor in developing skin cancer.

3) Occupational exposure to chemicals - many studies have centered around the worker's exposure to various chemicals and the resulting higher risks of getting cancer. Examples include exposure to petroleum distillates, vinyl chloride in the manufacture of PVC plastics, arsenic compounds, and benzene in those working with paints, varnishes, glues, etc.

4) Prolonged irritation - chronic irritation of localized areas of tissue is thought by many scientists to be involved in the formation of certain types of cancer. For example, cancer of the lip in pipe smokers seems to be associated with long-term irritation of the tissues in this area.

5) Viruses - since the early 1900's scientists have shown that viruses are involved in cancer development in lower animals such as mice, chickens, and rabbits. The role of viruses in human cancer is less well known, but studies in recent years are providing more and more evidence concerning the implication of viruses. The Epstein-Barr virus, which causes mononucleosis in humans, has been associated with a particular form of lymphoma occurring in Africa. However, it is also believed that this particular lymphoma occurs in patients whose immune system is already weakened by attacks of endemic malaria. Also, there is strong evidence in recent years that sexually transmitted viruses are involved in causing cervical cancer in women.

6) Hormones - the activity of certain hormones is also thought to be involved in the development of some tumors in the body. For example, many studies have pointed to the involvement of certain sex hormones in

developing breast cancer in women and prostate cancer in men. Hormone therapy is currently of great interest to scientists working on treatments for certain hormone-dependent tumors. Also, many cases are on file of women who at one time received certain hormone therapies during pregnancy in an effort to avoid miscarriages, but the hormone had the adverse effect of causing vaginal cancer in the daughters of these women.

Embalming Implications Associated With Tumors

Embalmers need to be aware of some important post-mortem conditions which are often associated with tumors of various types. One of these common post-mortem conditions is **emaciation.** Due to the chronic, long-term nature of most cancers, many patients will lose considerable body mass during the course of their disease, and considerable emaciation is quite likely to occur. The embalmer must take this emaciation into consideration when choosing his/her arterial fluids, selecting those which will best fill out and moisturize the tissues, restoring them to a natural appearance. In addition, emaciation may require additional treatments such as the use of tissue builder in areas of the face which appear abnormally shallow or sunken. The term **cachexia** is closely related to emaciation, and refers to a state of general ill health, malnutrition, and wasting away.

Discolorations are also often present in the tissues affected by tumors. These discolorations may require supplemental treatments to help bleach the area, such as compresses soaked with appropriate chemicals, or the hypodermic injection of bleaching agents into the area. In addition, cosmetic agents may be required to cover over persisting discolorations after other embalming techniques have been employed.

Hemorrhage as a result of damaged vessels is also a frequent complication associated with tumors. It should be anticipated that tumors have already destroyed and weakened many blood vessels in their vicinity, and that the increased pressure which accompanies routine arterial injection can result in the rupture of additional vessels, thus aggravating the problem of fluid distribution in the area around and beyond the tumor site.

Tissue deformation is another problem which often accompanies tumors. By the very nature of the disease, cancer often results in destruction and deformation of surrounding tissues. When these tissues are near the surface, particularly in the area of the face, they are likely to require additional care by the embalmer. Excision of tumors and associated necrotic tissue may be required, combined with supplemental embalming treatments such as compresses and hypodermic injection to assure proper preservation and disinfection of the affected areas. In addition, restorative treatments such as deep wound filling and waxing may be necessary to restore normal surface contour.

Tumors are also likely to result in **extravascular obstruction** to the flow of embalming fluid through the vessels. Even if a tumor is not malignant, it may well have the effect of putting pressure on surrounding vessels, thus resulting in partial or total occlusion of these vessels, and lack of fluid distribution beyond the point of the tumor. In cases such as this, multiple injection points may be necessary to assure the proper saturation of bodily tissues with embalming chemicals.

Chapter Six
DISEASES OF THE BLOOD

Anatomy Review

The liquid portion of blood is called plasma, which consists of water (about 92%), plus fibrin, and various salts and proteins. Suspended in blood plasma are the three main types of blood cells or corpuscles. Red blood cells (erythrocytes), which serve to carry oxygen to the tissues of the body and remove carbon dioxide, are the most numerous of the blood cells. There are about 4.5 to 5,000,000 of them per cubic millimeter of blood. White blood cells (leukocytes) are important in the body's defense mechanisms, performing such functions as phagocytosis and antibody formation. There are five main types of leukocytes, including neutrophils, basophils, eosinophils, lymphocytes, and monocytes. The number of white cells generally ranges from about 5,000 to 9,000 per cubic millimeter of blood. Platelets (thrombocytes) are blood cells which are involved in the process of clot formation. They are normally present in numbers of about 300,000 per cubic millimeter of blood.

Anemia

Anemia is a term whose literal meaning would be "no blood", so it is an example of a word which is actually used somewhat differently than its literal meaning indicates. In reality, anemia refers to a decrease in the number of red blood cells and/or hemoglobin. Any significant decrease in the number of red blood cells, or the hemoglobin they contain, will in turn result in a diminished supply of oxygen to the tissues of the body. Anemias are often characterized by weakness, fatigue, shortness of breath upon exertion, and lightheadedness. All of these can be attributed to the lower than normal supply of oxygen being delivered to the bodily tissues.

Two main groups of anemias are often identified, including the **primary** anemias, which are those diseases involving a decreased production of red blood cells, and **secondary** anemias, which involve an increased loss or destruction of red cells. In addition to this general classification, a determination is often made concerning the size of the red cell (normal, larger than normal, or smaller than normal), and the amount of hemoglobin it contains (normal amount, more than normal, or less than normal). A combination of these factors is often important in making a diagnosis concerning the exact type of anemia which a patient may be suffering from.

Pernicious anemia is one of decreased production usually associated with older age. It may be thought of as a deficiency disease, as it results from a lack of Vitamin B12 being absorbed from the digestive tract. Vitamin B12 is necessary and important for the normal development and maturation of cells in the body, including red blood cells. This disease may be a result of a diet lacking in Vitamin B12, or a deficiency in hydrochloric acid which is secreted by the mucous lining of the stomach, and is necessary for the absorption of Vitamin B12 molecules into the bloodstream. In addition to the general symptoms of anemia, pernicious anemia is often characterized by a smooth, red, painful tongue, and damage to cells in the nervous system, causing various neurologic disorders.

Another primary anemia is called **aplastic anemia**, which, as its name implies (a = none, plasia = formation), is characterized by a virtual stoppage of blood cell production in the bone marrow. The exact cause of aplastic anemia is not known, but it is thought that some cases are related to certain drugs and chemical agents, radiation, and other factors which may affect the normal hemopoietic function of the bone marrow.

Besides chronic hemorrhage, which can result in severe anemia, there are several other examples of secondary anemias, or those resulting in increased destruction of red blood cells. Secondary anemias are sometimes referred to as **hemolytic anemias.**

Sickle-cell anemia is a hemolytic anemia which results from a genetic defect in the manufacture of hemoglobin. The disease is characterized by an abnormal, crescent-shaped red blood cell, which is less functional as an oxygen carrier. These abnormal cells, referred to as "sickle-cells", are also more likely to cause thrombosis, and to be subjected to phagocytosis due to their unnatural shape and appearance. The genetic defect of sickle-cell anemia is confined largely to people of African descent, and may be transmitted by both males and females, with the most severe cases occurring in people who are homozygous for the trait, meaning they inherited the defective gene from each parent.

Erythroblastosis fetalis, or hemolytic disease of the newborn, is another example of a secondary anemia. This condition is basically a problem of blood incompatibility between a mother and her unborn fetus. The problem occurs when a mother who is Rh- carries a child who is Rh+. If fetal red cells manage to enter the mother's bloodstream, which is most likely to happen at delivery, the mother's body forms antibodies against the Rh factor in the fetal blood. These antibodies can then cross the placental barrier and destroy the blood of an unborn fetus, or the blood of a fetus in a subsequent pregnancy if the mixing occurred at delivery. *(See Fig. 16)*

Erythroblastosis fetalis gets its name due to the fact that the bloodstream of an affected child contains an abundance of erythroblasts, or immature red blood cells, which were generated by the bone marrow in a furious effort to compensate for the hemolytic activity which is occurring. The disease used to have a high mortality rate, with survival being attributed to successful exchange transfusions of blood. However, more modern and preferable actions involve treatment of an Rh- mother with an immune serum, to keep her body from forming antibodies against the Rh+ blood type.

Leukemia and Leukocytosis

Leukocytosis refers to an increase in the number of circulating white blood cells, and is an important defense mechanism of the body when it occurs in a temporary, or transient, fashion. If we recall, a white cell count of 5-9,000 per cubic millimeter is normal, with counts much higher (30-50,000 or more) during times of infection. However, when the disease condition is over with, the white cell count returns to normal.

Leukemia is a malignancy of the hemopoietic tissues in the body, and is sometimes referred to as "cancer of the blood". It is characterized by a relatively permanent and massive leukocytosis, unlike the transient increase in white cells which serves a protective function in the body. In leukemia, the white cells which are being produced are immature forms, and the bone marrow is turning them out in tremendous numbers, up to 800,000 to 1,000,000 per cubic millimeter of blood! These leukemic cells effectively crowd out the other blood cells, preventing the normal maturation of red blood cells and platelets.

Leukemias are often categorized based on the specific type of white cell which is affected, and they may be either chronic or acute. The two main forms are lymphoid (lymphocytic) leukemia, which affects mainly the body's lymph nodes and is characterized by the presence of many small lymphocytes in the blood, lymph nodes, and bone marrow. Acute lymphocytic leukemia is the most common form of cancer in children. The other main form of leukemia is called myeloid (myelocytic) leukemia, and shows an increase in myeloid cells, or the precursor cells in the bone marrow from which other granulocytic white cells are normally formed.

Some of the common signs and symptoms of leukemia include a swollen spleen and lymph nodes, fever, weight loss, fatigue, joint pain, and a tendency to hemorrhage. When increased numbers of white cells crowd out the normal functioning of red cells, this leads to symptoms of anemia, and the decreased number of platelets which can also result predisposes to abnormal bleeding in various parts of the body.

Whereas leukocytosis refers to an increase in the number of white cells, **leukopenia** would indicate a decrease in white blood cells. Various drugs, and conditions which suppress the bone marrow activity, may result in leukopenia. For example, the infectious disease typhoid fever, an acute intestinal infection with severe toxemia, often exhibits leukopenia as a sign, apparently because the bacillus causing the disease adversely affects bone marrow activity.

Polycythemia is a condition, as its name indicates (poly meaning many, cyte meaning cell, emia meaning blood), which is characterized by an increase in the number of blood cells in the body. Polycythemia vera is a serious form of polycythemia, characterized by overactive bone marrow which leads to an increase in all cellular elements, including red cells, which would be referred to as **erythrocytosis.** This condition results in increased blood viscosity, high blood pressure, and extra work on the heart. This extra-thick blood tends to congest in the various body organs and is predisposed to clotting.

Sometimes erythrocytosis may occur independent from any disease condition in the body. For instance, in an effort to compensate for a greater oxygen need, the body may produce extra red cells in order to carry the needed oxygen. People living in high altitudes where the oxygen content of the air is lower often experience this more controlled form of erythrocytosis, as do athletes such as long distance runners whose muscles regularly require increased oxygen amounts.

Bleeding Disorders

Hemophilia is an hereditary bleeding disorder, characterized by a greatly prolonged clotting time for blood. Someone with hemophilia may suffer from prolonged bleeding even from minor cuts or injuries. It is referred to as a sex-linked inherited disorder because the defective gene is transmitted on the X chromosome. It generally affects only males, but is transmitted by females.

Thrombocytopenia is a condition characterized by a decreased number of platelets, or thrombocytes, in the blood. Platelets are blood cells responsible for initiating the blood clotting process, and when they are present in less than normal amounts, definite tendencies to hemorrhage occur. When these hemorrhages occur as fairly widespread, spontaneous hemorrhages into the skin and mucous membranes, it is referred to as thrombocytopenic purpura, or just **purpura** (Latin meaning purple). The term **ecchymosis** is used to describe bruise-like patches of hemorrhage under the skin, and **petechiae** are small, red spots of hemorrhage, often described as "pin-point" hemorrhages. The word petechiae is from the Italian words for "flea bite".

In addition to thrombocytopenia leading to hemorrhages into the tissues, many serious febrile diseases such as meningitis and meningococcemia predispose to petechiae and ecchymotic hemorrhages.

Chapter Seven
DISEASES OF THE HEART AND VESSELS

Anatomy Review

The cardiovascular system consists of the heart, which serves as the pump to deliver blood to bodily tissues, and the blood vessels, which are the structures through which the blood moves throughout the body.

The heart is mainly a muscular organ, which is divided into three basic layers. The delicate inner lining is called the endocardium, the muscular walls are referred to as the myocardium, and the outer layer is the epicardium. The epicardium is actually the visceral portion of the pericardium, a double-layered sac which surrounds the heart.

The interior of the heart is divided into four chambers. The two upper chambers, or atria, serve as the receiving chambers, taking in blood which is returning from the various body parts. Blood leaving the atria passes through the right (tricuspid) and left (bicuspid/mitral) atrioventricular valves into the ventricles, which are the lower pumping chambers. As blood is pumped out of the ventricles, it passes through the pulmonary (right side) and aortic (left side) semilunar valves, enters the major arteries of the body, and is delivered to all bodily tissues. Blood which has reached the tissues of the body via the arteries then passes through the capillaries, continues on into the system of veins, and is returned to the heart.

That portion of the circulatory system which delivers deoxygenated blood from the right ventricle of the heart, over to the lungs for oxygen, and back to the left atrium is called pulmonary circulation. Systemic circulation involves delivery of oxygenated blood from the left ventricle of the heart to the tissues of the body and the return of deoxygenated blood to the right atrium.

Hypertrophy and Dilatation

Hypertrophy and **dilatation** (dilation) are two common conditions associated with various other diseases of the heart. Hypertrophy refers to an increase in the size of the heart (or part of the heart) due to an increase in the size of the muscle fibers. Hypertrophy usually occurs when an increased work load is put upon one or more of the heart chambers. For instance, if there is resistance to the flow of blood through the peripheral circulation, and the left ventricle has to work harder to force blood throughout the body, it is likely to hypertrophy. Or if there is chronic pulmonary disease, and the right ventricle has to work harder to pump blood through the lungs, then it may well hypertrophy. Disease of the heart valves also tends to result in hypertrophy, as proper function of these valves is important to a normal and orderly flow of blood through the heart, and consequently the entire body. (*See Fig. 17*)

Dilatation refers to the increase in the size of the heart, or a heart chamber, due to a stretching of the muscle fibers in the walls of the chamber. This usually occurs when the chamber becomes over-filled with blood on a regular basis. This may occur when heart valves are diseased and do not properly close, allowing a back-flow of blood into the chamber which it just left, or when there are openings in the atrial or ventricular septa, allowing blood to pass abnormally between the two atria or the two ventricles.

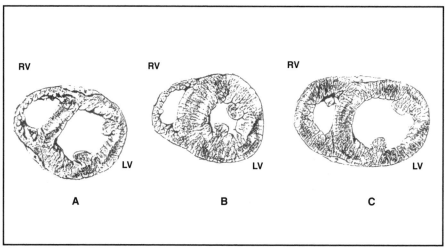

Cross section of the Heart showing hypertrophy and dilitation: Figure A shows a normal heart; Figure B shows a hypertrophied/thickened left ventricle due to prolonged pumping against high resistance in the systemic system; Figure C shows a hypertrophied/thickened right ventricle due to pumping against elevated pressure in the pulmonary system; and a dilated left ventricle.

Coronary Artery Disease

Coronary artery disease includes various conditions which affect the normal functioning of the coronary arteries, which are critical to the overall operation of the heart, as they are responsible for delivering the oxygen carrying blood to the heart muscle itself.

The term **occlusion** refers to a blocking or closing off of the coronary arteries from various causes. There are a number of conditions which may lead to coronary occlusion, including arteriosclerosis and atherosclerosis, which often results in a narrowing of the lumen (internal diameter) of the arteries. Thrombosis, or the formation of a blood clot, is another common cause of occlusion, especially in arteries which are already arteriosclerotic. In addition, the coronary arteries may become occluded by embolism, or blockage as a result of something which has floated into the arteries to partially or totally block the lumen. On occasion, diseases which result in spasms of muscle fibers in the walls of the heart may effectively cause occlusion of the coronary arteries.

The ischemia, or decreased blood flow, which results from coronary occlusion may lead to necrosis of heart tissue. This may be a slow process over time, with the formation of scar tissue in the heart, or it may be a rather sudden occurrence, in which case the common "heart attack" may occur. The scientific name for a heart attack is **myocardial infarction**, indicating death of heart tissue due to a lack of blood supply. The area of necrotic tissue which occurs is called an **infarct.** The severity of a heart attack depends on the particular artery involved and the degree to which it is occluded. *(See Fig. 18)* Even if a heart attack is not massive and fatal, it often results in permanent damage to certain areas of the heart, and may set the groundwork for additional heart disease in the future. *(See Fig. 19)*

Hypertensive Heart Disease

Hypertensive heart disease refers to the various changes which occur in the heart as a result of prolonged pumping against unusual resistance. The

40

resistance generally results from disease and narrowed peripheral blood vessels, and the heart, particularly the left ventricle, is required to pump harder and harder in order to meet the demand which is being placed upon it. Hypertrophy of the left ventricle occurs, and the heart may even wear out and fail as a result.

Hypertension, or high blood pressure, can be easily demonstrated by taking routine blood pressure readings. Blood pressure refers to the actual pressure exerted upon the walls of the arteries in the body, and it is reflected in a two-digit reading, such as 120/80. The first number is the systolic pressure, which indicates the arterial pressure which exists at the time the heart muscle is contracting and exerting its maximum pressure upon the vascular walls. The second number is the diastolic pressure, which reflects that pressure within the arteries when the ventricles of the heart are relaxing and filling back up with blood. Although blood pressure varies a lot from person to person, and even within the same individual at certain times, it is generally accepted that systolic blood pressure readings over 140 and/or diastolic readings over 90 are indicative of some form of high blood pressure.

Valvular Disease

When the valves in the heart are diseased, it stands to reason that their normal function will be impaired. The term **stenosis** refers to the narrowing of an opening or passageway, and stenosis is a common problem affecting the heart valves, particularly the atrioventricular valves. When a valve opening is stenotic, proper quantities of blood cannot pass through the valve, and the chamber behind the valve may hypertrophy in an effort to force blood through the narrowed opening.

Insufficiency and **incompetence** are terms also related to diseased valves, and they refer to the inability of a valve to close properly. Thus, when a valve does not properly close, it allows a back-flow, or regurgitation, of blood into the previous chamber of the heart. For example, mitral insufficiency could result in the left atrium undergoing dilatation as a result of a constant overfilling with blood. It not only is accommodating its normal volume of blood entering from the pulmonary veins, but also the blood which re-enters the chamber through an incompetent mitral valve when the left ventricle contracts.

Prolapse is a fairly common condition affecting the atrioventricular valves, especially the mitral valve. It is characterized by one or more of the cusps of the heart valve turning backwards into the atrium upon ventricular systole.

Besides congenital defects, two conditions which commonly cause stenosis and incompetence in the heart valves are rheumatic heart disease, which we will discuss shortly, and bacterial infections. **Bacterial endocarditis,** or inflammation of the inner lining of the heart, can have serious effects on the rather delicate valves in the heart. Bacterial infections do damage to the valves, causing swelling, ulceration, thrombosis, adhesions, and eventual scarring. These rigid, thickened, and scarred valves are in turn stenotic and incompetent.

Endocarditis may be an acute, fulminating disease, where the heart valves and endocardium are rapidly destroyed and death occurs within days or weeks, or it may be sub-acute. Sub-acute bacterial endocarditis (SBE) is characterized by chronic thrombi called vegetations which occur on the valves. *(See Fig. 20)*

41

These thrombi often break loose and become infected emboli which lodge in other vital organs such as the brain and kidneys. Endocarditis most commonly occurs as a focal infection which spreads from another body area. It is often associated with such procedures as tooth extractions and tonsillectomies. *Streptococcus pyogenes* and *Staphylococcus aureus* are two organisms which commonly cause endocarditis.

Another bacterial infection which commonly affects the heart is syphilis, which is caused by *Treponema pallidum*. The later stages of syphilis are characterized by damage to the aorta and aortic valve, often resulting in aneurisms and aortic insufficiency.

Besides the endocardium, the other heart layers are also subject to infection from various organisms. When the outer sac around the heart is inflamed it is called **pericarditis,** and inflammation of the heart muscle itself would be referred to as **myocarditis.**

Rheumatic Heart Disease

Rheumatic fever is a febrile, systemic disease which normally follows an attack of tonsillitis or strep throat caused by hemolytic streptococci. It is sometimes referred to as an immunological disease because it is interpreted as an allergic reaction to the previous strep infection. The antigen-antibody reaction which occurs tends to cause inflammation of all layers of the heart, as well as causing a variable arthritis. This disease tends to be a chronic one, with repeated acute attacks over the years.

The heart damage which results from rheumatic fever is referred to as **rheumatic heart disease**. Characteristically, the connective tissues within the heart and its lining endocardium are damaged, causing the formation of small nodules called **Aschoff's bodies**, which eventually develop into scar tissue. The most noticeable effects of this scarring are apparent on the heart valves, especially the mitral valve. When the mitral valve becomes thickened, rigid, and scarred, stenosis occurs, followed by atrial dilatation and a predisposition toward thrombosis. Other irregularities in the normal functioning of the heart also result over the long term, with all of these conditions often resulting in serious, chronic heart disease.

Fortunately rheumatic heart disease is not as serious a problem today as it used to be some years ago. A lot of this decreased incidence of the disease is attributed to better and more frequent use of antibiotics to control the streptococcal infections which predispose to rheumatic fever.

Congestive Heart Failure

Congestive heart failure is a general term given to the condition in which the heart is diseased and not able to adequately pump blood to meet the needs of the body. As a result of high blood pressure, arteriosclerosis, myocardial infarctions, etc., the heart's capacity is diminished and the entire body may suffer. Other terms similar to congestive heart failure used to describe a functionally weakened heart are myocardial insufficiency and cardiac decompensation. **Cardiomyopathy,** which is often associated with congestive heart failure, simply refers to disease of the heart muscle. Besides being associated with congestive heart failure, it may accompany such conditions as infectious diseases, hypertrophy of the heart chambers, or chronic alcoholism.

Congenital Heart Disease

Many heart conditions are congenital as opposed to acquired diseases. Some of the more common congenital heart conditions include those which involve septal defects, or defects in the walls separating the two atria or the two ventricles. Small openings between these chambers may be of little consequence, but larger ones can have serious, life threatening effects.

One of the main problems which results from septal defects is the mixing of blood between the left and right sides of the heart. As blood pressure is normally greater on the left side, these defects often result in oxygenated blood being shunted through the opening into the right side of the heart, resulting in excess blood being present in these chambers. This in turn can result in hypertrophy and dilatation of the right ventricle and the right atrium. Cyanosis is not usually present, unless cardiac failure occurs, because deoxygenated blood is not being added to the oxygenated left side of the heart. However, greater and greater stress is put upon the pulmonary circulation over time, which may result in eventual heart failure.

Septal defects may be the result of improper development of the walls in the heart, which accounts for most of the more serious problems, or failure of the fetal foramen ovale to properly close after birth. The foramen ovale is the normal opening which exists in the atrial septum of a fetus, allowing blood to pass from the right atrium directly into the left atrium and by-pass the non-functioning pulmonary system.

Another common congenital heart defect is called **patent** (Latin meaning open) **ductus arteriosus**, which means that the opening between the pulmonary artery and the aorta fails to close. The ductus arteriosus allows blood being pumped from the right ventricle to enter the aortic arch, as it does not need to enter the lungs for oxygenation in an unborn child. As with septal defects, a patent ductus arteriosus will result in a mixing of systemic and pulmonary blood. In addition to causing extra work for the right side of the heart, these defects predispose to infections and thrombosis occurring at the margins of the openings. Therefore, it is usually preferable to surgically repair these defects in order to avoid greater problems in the future.

Some heart defects are of such a nature that they allow for de-oxygenated blood from the right side of the heart to be shunted into the systemic circulation, in which case cyanosis, or a bluish discoloration of the skin, may be an obvious sign. Babies born with heart defects which allow for this form of blood mixing are often referred to as "blue babies".

Diseases of Vessels

Arteriosclerosis is a degenerative condition in which the arteries of the body become hardened, thickened, and inelastic as a result of the deposition of calcium in their walls. Many of the larger and important vessels such as the aorta, coronary arteries, and cerebral arteries, also tend to be affected by the formation of fatty deposits, called **plaques,** on the tunica intima of the vessels. The formation of these intimal plaques is referred to as **atherosclerosis,** and along with hardening of the arteries, results in one of the main health problems afflicting the human body. The end result of these degenerative processes in the arteries of the body is decreased blood flow to crucial areas. Arteries whose walls are hardened and lined with fatty deposits result in high blood pressure, thrombosis, ischemia, and weakened vessels predisposed to rupturing. *(See Fig. 21)*

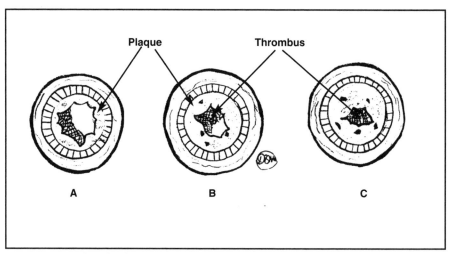

*Gradual occlusion of a vessel as a result of plaque
formation and thrombosis*

Although exact causes and reasons for these arterial diseases are not known, many factors have been implicated in their development. Among these are age, stress, smoking, lack of exercise, and diet, especially fat and cholesterol intake.

Aneurysm is a term which refers to a localized weakening and dilation of an artery wall. The main danger from an aneurysm is that it may rupture and result in hemorrhage, and depending on its location, this could be serious and even fatal. Rupture of cerebral aneurysms is a common cause of stroke, and syphilis is known to cause aneurysms of the aorta, which would certainly be serious if breakage were to occur on this major vessel.

There are several main types of aneurysm which are often identified. The first is called a **saccular** aneurysm, which is a bulging, sac-like dilation on the wall of an artery. Secondly, an aneurysm which results in a "tubular" swelling around the entire circumference of an artery is referred to as **fusiform.** The third type is called **dissecting** and is characterized by a weakening and separation between the walls of an artery, which may allow blood to make its way between layers of the vessel wall.

Arteritis refers to inflammation involving an artery, which may be a primary disease, or associated with various other conditions, such as rheumatic fever and various bacterial infections.

When the veins of the body become inflamed, it is referred to as **phlebitis.** Often closely associated with phlebitis is thrombosis, and when the two occur together, the condition is called thrombophlebitis. This condition most commonly occurs in the lower extremities.

Varicose veins, or **varices,** are those veins which become dilated and tortuous. They often form when the return of blood flow toward the heart is impeded. In addition to hereditary factors, conditions which predispose to varicose veins are standing or sitting for extended periods, pregnancy, tumors, and heart failure.

If we recall the anatomy of veins, particularly in the lower extremities, they contain valves which help the return of blood flow against gravity. When veins become swollen with blood, their valves become incompetent, and fail to prevent the back-flow of blood. Consequently, this magnifies the problem of blood stagnating and collecting in the veins. Blood which collects in veins,

44

and does not keep moving in the intended fashion, is predisposed to thrombus formation, and the swollen, knotty veins are also subject to mechanical injury and hemorrhage.

Besides the lower extremities, another common site for varices to occur is in the area of the rectum and anal canal. Varicose veins of this area are referred to as **hemorrhoids.**

Predisposing Factors in Cardiovascular Disease

Medical science has provided numerous studies over the years to help identify some of the more important factors involved in disease of the cardiovascular system. While not all research agrees on the exact nature and influence which various factors impart, there are some fairly well accepted generalities which should be mentioned when considering cardiovascular disease.

Following is a list of some major factors affecting the health of the cardiovascular system:

1) Heredity - An important question asked by doctors when taking medical histories is the occurrence of heart disease in the patient's family. Heredity seems to be a strong influence in many cardiovascular diseases.

2) Obesity - Carrying extra weight is known to put extra work upon the heart, and weight loss is a common part of many heart patient's overall treatment.

3) Diet - A healthy diet, low in fats and cholesterol, is another recommendation to help avoid cardiovascular disease. Atherosclerosis and hypertension are closely associated with our long-term dietary intake.

4) Diabetes - Diabetes mellitus, or sugar diabetes, is a disease which can have serious adverse effects upon the cardiovascular system. The disease is often characterized by vascular damage and occlusion, atherosclerosis, and possibly even gangrene, especially in the extremities.

5) Other social factors, such as stress, smoking, and alcohol and drug abuse are known to predispose to cardiovascular disease. Control of these factors can greatly improve the prognosis of a patient with heart disease.

Embalming Considerations in Cardiovascular Disease

Diseases of the cardiovascular system are of great concern to the embalmer, as they often have a direct impact upon the ultimate success of the embalming operation. Many of the diseases discussed in this chapter, as well as the chapter on diseases of the blood, result in intravascular resistance to the flow of embalming fluid. These various diseases which damage the vascular walls, narrow the lumen of a vessel, lead to easy rupture of fragile vessels, and predispose to thrombosis and increased blood viscosity, all pose valid concerns for the professional embalmer.

Pre-injection and co-injection chemicals are often required for their anti-coagulating abilities. Regardless of the strength of arterial chemicals which case analysis dictates, careful control of injection pressure and rate of flow of the arterial solution should be maintained. Rupture of fragile vessels and swelling of the tissues can result from careless use of excessive pressure and rate of flow during the embalming operation. Intravascular difficulties will most often require multiple injection points in order to assure the best possible distribution of fluid throughout the body. It is highly unlikely that a body which exhibits widespread arteriosclerosis, for example, can be properly embalmed through a single injection point.

In addition, careful raising and handling of arteriosclerotic vessels is an important consideration. The embalmer may wish to consider a longitudinal or triangular type of incision, as opposed to the more common transverse incision, in order to avoid breakage of particularly fragile vessels. Care should be taken in tying off weak vessels to avoid their further damage.

Chapter Eight
DISEASES OF THE DIGESTIVE SYSTEM

Anatomy Review

The digestive system is responsible for the intake of nutrients and the elimination of waste products from the body. The mouth is the beginning point of the digestive system, where the action of chewing begins the mechanical breakdown of food products, and saliva is added to begin the chemical aspect of digestion. Upon swallowing, food passes through the pharynx, the esophagus, and into the stomach. Here the food is further mixed with digestive juices to prepare it for eventual absorption in the small intestine, which it will next enter.

The small intestine is subdivided into three main segments, called the duodenum, the jejunum, and the ileum. By the time food has passed through the small intestine, it has been chemically and mechanically digested to the point that most of the nutrients present have been absorbed into the bloodstream.

Upon leaving the small intestine, the residual products in the digestive tract enter the large intestine, where much of the water is removed prior to the elimination of waste products in the form of feces. The cecum is the first part of the large intestine, followed by the colon, rectum, and anal canal.

The entire digestive tract, from the mouth to the anal canal, is sometimes referred to as the alimentary canal. Accessory organs of digestion, which are also important in the digestive process, include such structures as the tongue, teeth, salivary glands, pancreas, and the liver.

Diseases of the Mouth and Throat Area

Due to the fact that the mouth is a natural reservoir for a multitude of bacteria and viruses, many inflammations and infections can affect the oral cavity. **Stomatitis** refers to inflammation of the mouth, and it can take many forms. Besides infection from pathogens, inflammation of the mouth may result from such things as trauma, chemical irritation, burns, tobacco, etc.

Aphthous (Greek meaning ulcer) stomatitis is a common condition characterized by the formation of tiny white ulcers which form at the base of the gums, lips, and cheeks. These ulcers are commonly referred to as "canker sores". These sores often appear for unapparent reasons, but many times are associated with mechanical injury to the mucosa, dietary disturbances, hormonal activity, and possibly even genetics.

Other organisms causing inflammation of the oral cavity include *Candida albicans*, the fungus which causes thrush, and Herpes simplex I, a viral infection commonly seen as cold sores or fever blisters. *Treponema pallidum*, the causative agent of syphilis, can also lead to inflammatory lesions in the mouth, referred to as mucous patches, during the secondary stage of the disease.

Closely associated with stomatitis are **gingivitis** or inflammation of the gums, and **glossitis,** or inflammation of the tongue.

Tonsillitis refers to inflammation of the tonsils, which are masses of lymphoid tissue located in the walls of the oral pharynx. This is a common form of infection, usually caused by streptococcal organisms. Chronic cases of the disease, with the swelling which accompanies it, may require removal of the tonsils to prevent blockage of the airways. However, the development of modern antibiotics has greatly reduced the need for tonsillectomies in recent years.

Pharyngitis involves inflammation of the pharynx, or throat, and may be a primary infection such as strep throat or diphtheria, or a complication of other infections such as rhinitis, sinusitis, or influenza.

47

Diseases of the Esophagus and Stomach

The esophagus may also be affected by inflammation, in which case it is referred to as **esophagitis.** Sometimes esophagitis is a result of the regurgitation of stomach acid through the cardiac sphincter valve, resulting in a chemical irritation of the mucosa lining the esophagus.

Besides inflammation, the esophagus is often affected by stenosis or stricture, which indicates an abnormal narrowing of the organ. Serious infections or chemical irritation, which may lead to the formation of scar tissue within the esophagus, may lead to stricture. Another common cause of narrowing of the esophagus is tumors which develop, either within the lumen of the organ, or outside the esophagus, resulting in pressure being placed on its muscular walls.

Gastritis, which refers to inflammation of the stomach, may be caused by many things, most commonly bacterial and viral infections, and chemical irritants such as coffee, alcohol, aspirin, and tobacco. Hemorrhage from the lining of the stomach is a danger of severe gastritis, and often accompanies chronic alcoholism. The vomiting of blood from the stomach, often associated with gastritis, is referred to as **hematemesis.**

An ulcer is a localized area of necrosis on the skin or mucous membrane. Dead tissue is sloughed off, often resulting in a hole or crater at the site. Ulcers which occur in the stomach and duodenum are referred to as **peptic ulcers,** deriving their name from the digestive enzyme known as pepsin, which is secreted by the mucosal lining of the stomach. Secretion of an excess amount of gastric juices is usually associated with the formation of peptic ulcers.

The main danger to the patient with an ulcer is that hemorrhage may occur, and the resulting loss of blood may be severe. Also, in the more serious cases, ulcers may perforate through the wall of the stomach or intestine, allowing the contents of the digestive tract, including bacteria, to reach the abdominal cavity. *(See Fig. 22)* This can result in a serious and even fatal case of **peritonitis,** or infection of the lining membrane of the abdominal cavity.

In addition to hemorrhage and peritonitis, another after-effect of peptic ulcers, especially chronic ones, may be the formation of scar tissue during the inflammation process. As the pyloric area of the stomach, and the initial part of the duodenum, are the most common sites for these ulcers to occur, the formation of scar tissue in these areas may result in **pyloric stenosis.** This in turn can have adverse effects upon the normal passage of food products from the stomach into the small intestine.

Diseases of the Intestines

Inflammations of the intestinal tract are quite common, especially as a result of in-fection by various organisms. Inflammation of the small intestine is referred to as **enteritis,** and inflammation of the colon, the main portion of the large intestine, is called **colitis.** Inflammation of the rectum is referred to as **proctitis,** and **appendicitis** indicates inflammation of the vermiform appendix. *(See Fig. 23)*

As with peptic ulcers, a danger associated with intestinal infections, especially appendicitis, is perforation of the intestinal tract, followed by peritonitis. Appendicitis is usually an acute infection, and can be easily treated by surgical removal of the organ, but if rupture occurs before medical attention is received, the resulting peritonitis can be difficult to control and may even prove fatal.

In addition to the danger of perforation, intestinal infections such as colitis and dysentery can result in severe diarrhea, causing the body to become seriously dehydrated. The normal function of the colon is to absorb water and other essential elements through its walls and back into the bloodstream. Inflammation can adversely affect this function, resulting in loss of much needed water through the digestive system.

There are numerous organisms which can result in intestinal infections, some of which are normal flora found in the intestinal tract, and act as opportunists, only causing infection when conditions become right for them to overstep their normal boundaries and result in disease. Some common infections of the intestinal tract, and the organisms which cause them, include:

1) Amoebic dysentery - *Entamoeba histolytica*

2) Typhoid fever - *Salmonella typhi*

3) Bacillary dysentery - *Shigella* species

4) Tuberculosis - *Mycobacterium tuberculosis*

5) Food poisoning - *Staphylococcus aureus, Clostridium perfringens, and Clostridium botulinum*

6) Enteritis - *Escherichia coli*, & others

Occasionally the intestinal tract is affected by small, pouch-like structures which protrude into the walls of the intestine. These little sacs, somewhat akin to a saccular aneurysm on an artery, are referred to as diverticula. The condition of having one or more diverticula is called **diverticulosis.** *(See Fig. 24)* They are often asymptomatic, but may become impacted with fecal material and bacteria, causing inflammation referred to as **diverticulitis.**

The rectal area is commonly affected by varicose veins called **hemorrhoids.** Any condition which puts pressure on the veins in this area, or obstructs the outflow of blood from the pelvic cavity, may predispose to hemorrhoids. Such conditions as pregnancy, constipation, tumors, enlarged prostate glands, and liver conditions resulting in portal obstruction are often associated with hemorrhoids.

The term **hernia** refers to protrusion of an organ through the walls of the body cavity in which it is contained. Many forms of hernia occur, some of which are referred to as abdominal hernias, where a tear or weak spot develops in the musculature of the abdominal wall, and part of the peritoneum, or a loop of intestine, pushes out through this opening. Inguinal hernias, which occur in the groin area, are some of the most common forms. Umbilical hernias often occur in infants due to imperfect closure of the abdominal wall in the area where the umbilical cord was attached. Also, herniation of part of the stomach through the esophageal opening in the diaphragm is called a hiatal hernia.

A main danger associated with hernias is the fact that the blood supply to the intestine may be pinched off, resulting in necrosis of tissue and possible gangrene. In addition, the intestine may become obstructed, resulting in interference with the passage of its contents.

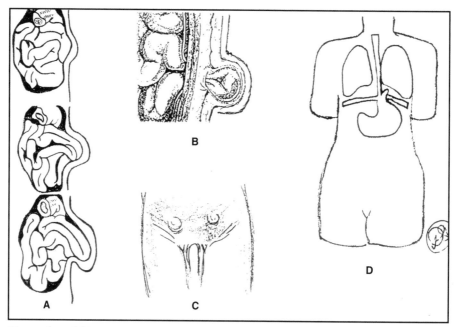

Examples of Hernias: A) Enlarging hernia (top to bottom) on lower abdominal wall; B) Side view of incarcerated hernia; C) Anterior view of hernias on lower abdominal wall; D) Hiatal hernia, with stomach protruding through diaphragm

In addition to obstruction of the intestinal tract from hernias, other forms of obstruction may occur. Following is a list of some common conditions which may lead to intestinal obstruction:

1) Tumors, either from within, or from outside, causing external pressure

2) Paralysis - lack of blood or nerve supply to a part of the intestine can paralyze it, resulting in decreased peristalsis, which serves to move the contents along

3) Volvulus - a twisting of a loop of intestine

4) Intussusception - a slipping, or telescoping, of one segment of intestine into the succeeding one *(See Fig. 25)*

5) Adhesions - the intestine may be distorted and partially obstructed when scar tissue forms and loops of the bowel adhere together where they normally would not do so.

Diseases of the Liver, Gallbladder, and Pancreas

Hepatitis refers to inflammation of the liver, and the most common causes of hepatitis are several strains of viruses. **Hepatitis A**, also known as **infectious** hepatitis, is a form of infection usually transmitted via contaminated food and water supplies. It is usually less serious than some other forms of hepatitis, and the prognosis is normally good, often without permanent damage to the liver.

Hepatitis B, or **serum** hepatitis, is another form of hepatitis which is more likely to be transmitted through contaminated body fluids, such as blood or semen. The disease is often passed among drug addicts who share needles and syringes under unsanitary conditions. This form of hepatitis is of concern to health care workers and embalmers, as it can be contracted from inadvertent puncture wounds from needles, scalpel blades, and other instruments. Hepatitis B is usually more serious than Hepatitis A, often resulting in chronic hepatitis, and permanent liver damage. However, there is a commercially available vaccine to protect against Hepatitis B, and those workers, such as embalmers, who come into regular contact with blood and body secretions, are well advised to take advantage of the protection which is offered.

Other strains of viral hepatitis have also been identified, including type C, or Non-A non-B hepatitis. In addition, **toxic hepatitis** may result from the liver attempting to perform its normal function of detoxifying the bloodstream. Excess quantities of drugs or poisons which enter the bloodstream, and collect in the liver, may result in inflammation and damage to liver tissue.

Cirrhosis is a long-term degeneration of the functioning cells of the liver, with a proliferation of fibrous connective tissue and scarring. Cirrhosis is often associated with chronic alcoholism, but may also result from damage done by drugs, toxins, and previous viral or bacterial infections.

Due to the damage which is done to liver cells, and the loss of their normal function, numerous effects of cirrhosis are often seen, either as ante-mortem or post-mortem conditions. Included in these are **jaundice,** due to the build-up of bile pigments in the bloodstream, and **ascites,** or edema of the abdominal cavity. When blood cannot properly flow through the damaged liver, passive hyperemia occurs in the portal system, and results in the collection of edematous fluid. In addition, **edema** occurs in other parts of the body because the liver has failed to produce some of its normal proteins such as albumin, which affects the permeability of the vascular walls, allowing fluid to leak out into the tissues. Toxins also build up in the blood because the liver is unable to remove them as it normally would.

Hemorrhage also tends to be a complication of cirrhosis, due partially to the great pressure put upon the veins in the portal system, and partially because the liver is not producing adequate blood proteins essential to the blood clotting process.

The gallbladder, which is the sac-like structure attached to the liver for the purpose of storing bile, may become inflamed, in which case it is referred to as **cholecystitis.** Cholecystitis is often associated with the formation of gallstones, which is called **cholelithiasis.** Gallstones may block the passageways for bile, causing it to collect and concentrate in the gallbladder, resulting in irritation and inflammation. *(See Fig. 26)* Gallstones often form when substances normally present in bile precipitate out of solution, forming hardened stones of varying size. *(See Fig. 27)* Blockages by gallstones in the bile ducts may also cause bile to back up in the liver, spill over into the bloodstream, and cause jaundice. If the bile ducts themselves become inflamed, it is referred to as **cholangitis.**

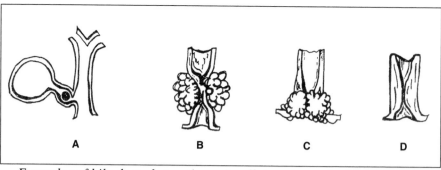

Examples of bile duct obstruction: a) gallstone in cystic duct; b) tumor pressing on duct from outside; c) tumor growing within duct; d) stricture

Pancreatitis involves inflammation of the pancreas, and may be either acute or chronic. Sometimes it is associated with gallstone blockages, where bile cannot enter the duodenum and is forced into the pancreatic duct, causing irritation of pancreatic tissues. Pancreatitis is also often associated with chronic alcoholism.

Many cases of pancreatitis are idiopathic, or of unknown cause. Occasionally pancreatic enzymes, which are intended for normal digestive processes, become active within the pancreas and begin to digest the tissues of the organ itself. This can lead to necrosis and hemorrhage, and severe cases of pancreatitis may prove fatal.

Tumors can and do affect nearly all parts of the digestive system. *(See Fig. 28)* Carcinomas affecting the epithelial lining of the alimentary canal are the most common form of cancer in the digestive system. Carcinomas occur frequently in the lips and mouth area, the pharynx, esophagus, and the stomach. The small intestine is less frequently affected by cancer than the colon and rectum. Colon and rectal cancers are the most prevalent of all digestive system cancers, and are a leading cause of death among cancer patients in the United States. *(See Fig. 29)*

In addition to malignant tumors, the intestinal tract is commonly affected by **polyps,** which are normally benign tumors which develop on mucous membranes. *(See Fig. 30)* They are also formed on the mucous membranes lining the respiratory tract, especially the nasal passages. Although polyps are generally benign, they may turn malignant, and should be watched by a doctor for changes indicating a pre-cancerous condition.

Embalming Considerations

Diseases of the digestive system present the embalmer with a number of concerns, some of which are unique to this particular system, and some which are more general in nature. Generally speaking, infections of the digestive tract can lead to such problems as **dehydration, rapid blood coagulation**, and **rapid decomposition**, just like other febrile diseases affecting the body. Edema, especially **ascites,** also accompanies many digestive diseases, as was mentioned under the discussion of cirrhosis. Each of these conditions requires the embalmer to closely evaluate the amount, strength, and type of embalming chemicals to be used. For example, edema cases will predispose to a higher secondary dilution of arterial and cavity chemicals, infectious diseases, with their high bacterial activity, may indicate the need for a stronger germicidal chemical, and dehydration may call for larger volumes of milder solutions.

Of particular concern to the embalming operator is the occurrence of jaundice, which often accompanies disease of the liver and gall bladder. Any time the embalmer observes that jaundice is present, or even suspects its presence, special jaundice fluids should be used for arterial injection, with extra care being given to the task of removing the yellow discoloration without promoting the development of a deeper green discoloration.

An additional concern with many digestive system diseases is that of abdominal distention which may result from both edema and the collection of gases in the digestive tract. This increased distention created within the abdominal area puts pressure on the major vessels, impairing both arterial distribution of embalming solutions and venous drainage of body fluids. Such distention may indicate additional injection and drainage points in order to assure thorough distribution of fluid to the tissues.

Pressure within the abdominal cavity may also pre-dispose to purge from the nose and mouth, which in turn will require that extra steps be taken to prevent additional problems from occurring. It may be necessary to puncture or incise the intestines to relieve the pressure, and applying massage cream to the lips and face will help prevent dehydration as a result of acidic purge flowing over the tissues in these areas.

Chapter Nine

DISEASES OF THE RESPIRATORY SYSTEM

Anatomy Review

The respiratory system is responsible for providing a fresh supply of oxygen to the body's blood, and removing the waste gas called carbon dioxide. When we breath in, air passes through the nasal passages, into the pharynx (throat), enters the larynx (voicebox), then the trachea (windpipe), the bronchi, the bronchioles, and ends up in the air sacs of the lungs called alveoli.

It is in the lungs where the exchange of gases called external respiration occurs. Oxygen passes through the walls of the alveoli, into the surrounding capillaries, and is picked up by the red blood cells present in these capillaries. Carbon dioxide gas passes in the opposite direction, being given off by the red cells and entering the alveoli, to be eliminated from the body with each breath we exhale.

Surrounding each lung is a double-layered serous membrane called the pleura, which is a slick, lubricating membrane which helps to reduce friction from the constant expansion and contraction of the lungs within the chest cavity. The minimal space between the two layers of pleura is called the pleural cavity.

The respiratory tract is lined with a mucous membrane, which serves to moisten and warm inspired air, and to trap foreign particles and bacteria which may enter from the external environment. Also contained within this specialized respiratory epithelium are numerous hair-like projections called cilia, which provide a sweeping action to help prevent the entry of unwanted foreign particles and organisms.

Upper Respiratory Diseases

The **common cold**, sometimes referred to as **coryza**, is an acute viral infection of the upper respiratory tract. As we all know, a cold is characterized by nasal congestion, runny nose and eyes, and mild sore throat and fever. Being a viral disease, there is no cure for the common cold, and unfortunately an attack of the disease does not confer immunity against further occurrences. Actually, numerous strains of viruses have been identified which are implicated in causing colds.

The term **rhinitis** refers to inflammation of the nasal passages, which is always a big part of having a cold. If the paranasal sinuses are also involved in the infection, it would be referred to as **sinusitis.** As with many viral infections, a cold is often complicated by bacterial infections affecting the sinuses, throat, and even into the lower respiratory tract and lungs. Inflammation of the throat is called **pharyngitis,** and inflammation of the voicebox is called **laryngitis.**

Hay fever is a common upper respiratory problem, and is described as a form of allergy, characterized by watery and itchy eyes, a runny nose, and sneezing and coughing as a result of hypersensitivity to various grass and tree pollens. In someone who has hay fever, a reaction between antibodies present in their system and the specific antigen (pollen) causes the release of a substance called histamine from certain cells in the body. Histamine in turn causes the dilation of surrounding capillaries, which then become "leaky" and secrete excess plasma into the tissues. This edematous fluid is what's responsible for causing the congestion and runny noses associated with hay fever. Hence the common practice of taking antihistamines in an effort to block the action of histamines and reducing this congestion and watery mucous membranes.

Influenza, usually called the flu, is a common viral infection affecting the upper respiratory tract, and characterized by fever, chills, sore throat, runny nose, cough, and often muscle pain. A number of viruses can lead to influenza, and the disease is a highly contagious one, often occurring in epidemic form. Cases of the flu may be mild in nature, or severe and even fatal. During 1918-19 a worldwide pandemic of flu affected hundreds of millions of people, killing an estimated 15-20 million individuals! More recent epidemics have been considerably more mild than this episode, but those who are very young, the elderly, and otherwise weakened individuals are the most susceptible to more serious cases of the flu.

The greatest danger with flu cases is that the viral infection adversely affects the respiratory epithelium, which is an important bodily defense mechanism. When this line of defense is compromised, secondary bacterial invaders are able to work their way down the respiratory tract and lead to other serious infections such as bronchopneumonia.

Lower Respiratory Diseases

An infection of the trachea would be referred to as **tracheitis,** and inflammation of the bronchi is **bronchitis.** Bronchitis is a common disease, and as with the flu, is most serious in infants, the elderly, and the chronically ill. It often occurs after another upper respiratory infection, but may be a primary disease. Besides fever, chest pain, and difficulty breathing, it is characterized by a chronic cough, as patients with the disease attempt to clear excess mucous from the lining of the respiratory passageways. In addition to microbial causes, bronchitis may result from long term exposure to dusts, pollutants, and cigarette smoking. *(See Fig. 31)*

Asthma is a form of allergy characterized by hypersecretion of mucous and spasms of the bronchial muscles. Some people are overly sensitive to various antigens, such as animal hair or feathers, dusts, certain food products, and various other chemicals. These antigenic substances cause abnormal, spasmodic contractions of the musculature in the bronchial passageways. In addition, excess mucous is secreted by the respiratory mucosa, and as a result, the airways are narrowed, making breathing difficult. Asthma attacks are characterized by a "wheezing" sound from air passing through these obstructed airways.

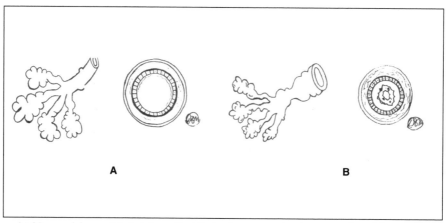

A) *Normal bronchiole/alveoli*   B) *Asthma results in constricted bronchioles with mucous build-up in the lumen causing obstruction*

Although there is no cure for asthma, various medications are available to lessen its symptoms and to help dilate the air passageways. Tests can be run to help determine what the offending antigens are, and avoidance of these substances can help reduce the incidence of asthmatic attacks. Besides direct contact with a particular antigen, attacks may be brought on by other factors such as emotional stress, infections, chemical irritants, and smoke.

Pneumonia, or **pneumonitis,** is an inflammation of the lungs, generally with the collection of inflammatory exudates in the alveoli. Pneumonia may be caused by many organisms, including viruses and various types of bacteria.

Lobar pneumonia is one of the more common forms of the disease, and is so named because the infection tends to be localized in one or two lobes of the lung. The affected lobe(s) is usually consolidated with a thick, fibrinous exudate, which makes respiration in that portion of the lung virtually impossible. The disease is most often a primary one, with the organism *Streptococcus pneumoniae* causing a majority of the cases. Inflammation of the pleura, or the membranes surrounding the lungs, commonly accompanies lobar pneumonia. This **pleuritis,** or **pleurisy,** as it is called, results in severe pain upon breathing due to the fact that the inflamed membranes are rubbing against each other when the chest expands and contracts.

Cases of lobar pneumonia are often quite acute and severe, but respond well to antibiotic treatment, and are often resolved in a week to ten days with proper care.

Bronchial pneumonia, or **bronchopneumonia,** is the second main category of pneumonia, and is so named because it is primarily an inflammation of the bronchi and bronchioles, which can spread into the lungs. Unlike lobar pneumonia, bronchopneumonia tends to be more scattered throughout both lungs and the bronchi, occurring in spotty patches, and not consolidating in one or two lobes of the lung. *(See Fig. 32)* Like lobar pneumonia, it is often caused by the pneumococcus, but is also caused by other organisms such as staphylococcus and other streps. Bronchopneumonia is more often a secondary disease, and characteristically complicates other diseases such as whooping cough, measles, influenza, chronic bronchitis, and cancer. It is a common hospital acquired (nosocomial) infection, and can be a serious threat to patients who are in a weakened state from various other conditions. Bronchopneumonia often does not resolve as well as lobar pneumonia, and is predisposed to chronic recurrences.

As was mentioned earlier, pleuritis refers to inflammation of the pleura, and accompanies various other infectious diseases such as pneumonia, tuberculosis, and influenza. When inflammatory exudates which collect in the pleural cavity are purulent (containing pus) in nature, the condition may be referred to as **empyema** or **pyothorax.** If fluid is collecting in the pleural cavity, and it is more watery, or edematous in nature, it is referred to as **pleural effusion,** or **hydrothorax.** Unlike the pustular exudate associated with infections, hydrothorax is more likely to accompany circulatory disorders, such as heart failure, which produce generalized edemas.

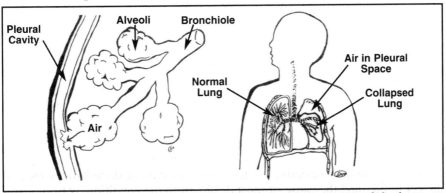

Atelectasis due to air entering pleural cavity after rupture of the lung

Other substances, such as blood and air, may also collect in the pleural cavities. **Hemothorax,** indicating a collection of blood, may accompany some infections, wounds, tumors, etc. Air in the pleural cavity is referred to as **pneumothorax,** and may result from penetrating wounds from the outside, or from ruptured alveoli in conditions such as tuberculosis or emphysema. Whenever substances such as blood, fluid, pus, or air collect in the pleural cavity, they put pressure on the lung and may cause it to collapse. The term **atelectasis** is given to the condition of having a collapsed lung. A lung may also collapse due to obstruction of a bronchus, as may occur from severe bronchitis or a tumor growing in the passageway. Air in the lung is absorbed, new air cannot enter to keep the lung inflated, and the lung collapses. Atelectasis may also be a congen-ital condition, in which the lungs fail to expand and aerate after birth.

Emphysema is a respiratory disease which can be described as a long term, chronic deterioration and destruction of lung tissue. It is not an infectious disease, but one which is normally associated with long term irritation of the respiratory passageways. It is often a complication of chronic bronchitis and other respiratory irritations, such as smoking and environmental pollutants.

Emphysema is characterized by the inability of normal external respiration to take place. The lungs stay filled with air high in carbon dioxide, and the patient experiences a suffocating feeling due to the inability to get enough oxygen into the lungs. This poor respiratory exchange is due to irritation and excess mucous production within the bronchi and bronchioles. The end result of the disease is a breakdown of the delicate walls of the alveoli, and a joining together of the tiny air sacs into much larger, functionless sacs called bullae. *(See Fig. 33)* These bullae may eventually rupture and allow air into the pleural cavity, leading to pneumothorax and atelectasis. Many emphysema patients show a characteristic "barrel chest" due to prolonged labored breathing, and constant, abnormal expansion of the chest.

Emphysema is truly a debilitating disease, as it causes great pain and distress for those suffering from it with each breath they take over the years.

The condition referred to as **chronic obstructive pulmonary disease (COPD)** is somewhat of an umbrella term encompassing the various conditions which cause long-term interference with the normal respiratory exchange of gases. Under this heading are included emphysema, chronic bronchitis, and bronchial asthma. Two or more of these conditions often co-exist, joining forces to obstruct the normal flow of oxygen and carbon dioxide into and out of the lungs, thus the general designation of COPD.

Along with these discussions of respiratory obstruction, it is important to mention the disease **cystic fibrosis.** This is a condition which affects several body systems, but particularly those with exocrine secretory functions, such as the pancreas and the sweat glands. Also, mucous membranes lining various body parts, including the respiratory tract, are generally affected.

Cystic fibrosis is often discussed along with diseases of the pancreas, and the name of the disease derives from the fact that excessively thick and sticky mucous secretions block the pancreatic ducts, and result in a dilation of glands into sac-like structures called cysts. These cysts may be converted into fibrous tissue, hence the name cystic fibrosis. The resulting lack of pancreatic digestive enzyme leads to severe dietary disturbances.

Although this disease derives its name from pancreatic disturbances, the real danger to life, and the cause of most deaths from the condition, is from respiratory obstruction which results from the thick and sticky mucous secretions of the membranes lining the air passageways to the lungs. In addition to blocking the flow of air into the lungs, this heavy mucous also traps bacteria and predisposes to serious respiratory infections.

Cystic fibrosis is an hereditary disease, normally affecting children. It is a result of a genetic disorder controlling the secretory functions of the glands. Although there is no cure for the disease, modern antibiotic treatments to prevent bacterial infections and respiratory therapy methods to help reduce congestion have somewhat improved the outlook of the condition in recent years.

Pneumoconiosis is another non-communicable, non-infectious condition affecting the lungs. It is a combination word meaning "lungs", "dust", and "pathological condition". It may be defined as infiltration and discoloration of the lungs due to prolonged inhalation of dust. The irritation caused by dust accumulation over the long term can lead to fibrosis and scarring of the lung tissue.

Pneumoconiosis is generally an occupational disease, with the actual type of dust identified in the name of the disease. For example, fine particles of silica, or stone dust, which are common hazards for workers in such areas as mining, rock-quarrying, and sandblasting, gives us the form of pneumoconiosis called **silicosis. Anthracosis,** from the word anthracite, which is a form of coal, refers to discoloration of the lungs due to coal dust. This condition is commonly known as "black lung" disease, and has been responsible for robbing the breath from coal miners for decades. Another example of pneumoconiosis is **asbestosis,** which involves the inhalation of asbestos fibers. Asbestos is a widely used product in industry, with literally hundreds of different applications.

Insulation and building products are two of the main areas of asbestos usage, and the manufacture and use of these products has been widely associated with many individuals inhaling fibers which are harmful to the respiratory system. Not only are they irritants, but in recent years a definite link has been shown between asbestosis and lung cancer.

Tuberculosis is a serious infectious and communicable disease caused by the bacillus *Mycobacterium tuberculosis*. The virulence of the bacillus is enhanced by its cell wall, which contains a high lipid content, providing the organism with a somewhat "waxy" coat which helps protect it against germicides and adverse environmental factors. The bacillus can exist for long periods of time in dried specks of sputum or blood, and be spread in these dust particles to inhabit and infect new hosts.

Pulmonary tuberculosis, affecting the lungs, is the most common form of the disease, but it may affect any body organ, especially the brain, kidneys, intestines, bones, and skin. It is normally contracted via the respiratory route, from droplet spray or contaminated hands and fomites. The disease often spreads through the blood and lymph vessels, forming tiny, widely dispersed foci of infection resembling millet seeds. This resemblance to millet seeds gives this form of the disease its designation of **miliary** tuberculosis.

After a primary infection with the TB bacillus, antibodies are produced and the body becomes sensitized, or allergic, to reinfection by the organism. Often a primary infection is controlled and arrested by the body's defenses, leaving only small areas of fibrous tissue where damage was done by the infection. Due to the fact that the body is sensitized to the

TB bacillus, and the nature of the reaction which occurs as a result of re-infection, chronic TB is characterized by the formation of lesions called **tubercles.** In its fight against the bacillus, the body forms a fibrous capsule around the infection site. As the tubercle grows in size, pressure is put upon surrounding capillaries, and circulation is impaired in the area. As a result of this circulatory interruption, plus the destructive effect of the bacilli, a characteristic form of necrotic tissue forms within the tubercle. This material resembles a soft, cheesy mass, and is referred to as **caseation** (Latin meaning cheese) necrosis.

Tubercles may undergo a number of changes throughout the course of the disease. Sometimes the contents of the tubercle become liquefied, resembling pus, but without all of the characteristic signs of inflammation. When this happens, it may be referred to as a **cold abscess. Cavitation** occurs when the growth of a tubercle erodes the walls of an adjacent bronchus, and the contents are thrown off into the air passageway, leaving an empty cavity.

Hemorrhage is also often seen as a complication of TB. Tubercle formation can damage blood vessels, resulting in **hemoptysis,** or the spitting up of blood.

In addition to caseation necrosis, cavitation, cold abscess formation, and hemorrhage, patients with tuberculosis are likely to show considerable emaciation and dehydration due to the chronic, debilitating nature of the disease. The professional embalmer should take these considerations into account when deciding upon the proper method of treatment of a dead body infected with tuberculosis.

In the earlier part of this century, tuberculosis was a devastating disease which was invariably fatal if it proceeded beyond an undetected primary infection. Special hospitals, called TB sanitariums, were used to care for and keep terminal patients with the disease. With the advent of effective antibiotic therapy in recent decades, the incidence of the disease has dropped dramatically in this country. However, TB remains a serious infectious disease, and studies have shown it to be making a strong comeback in many parts of the country. Drug resistant strains of the organism are evolving, and many cases of the disease are seen associated with immune suppressed individuals such as AIDS patients.

Carcinoma of the lung is one of the leading forms of cancer in the United States, and is the number one cause of death among male cancer patients in this country. *(See Fig. 34)* Lung cancer can be either primary at the site, or as a result of metastasis from other areas in the body. In addition, lung cancers may spread to other body areas, including the regional lymph nodes, brain, adrenal glands, liver, and the bones. One of the most common types of neoplasm to affect the respiratory tract is called bronchogenic carcinoma, due to its primary localization in one of the main bronchi. This type of tumor develops from the epithelium in the respiratory tract, and may even grow to the point that occlusion of the affected bronchi results. This may in turn result in atelectasis, or collapse, of the corresponding lung. Recurrent infections and abscesses of the area around and beyond the obstruction are also important complications associated with carcinomas of the lung.

Although all causes of lung cancer are not known, most scientists believe that cigarette smoking is directly related to the development of lung cancer. While not all smokers get cancer, and not all lung cancer patients are smokers, studies show a definite and dramatic increase in cases of lung cancer in smokers, compared to the general population. In addition to smoking, it is thought that other constant respiratory irritants, such as polluted air, can predispose to lung cancers.

Embalming Considerations

Several post-mortem conditions of concern to the embalmer have already been mentioned in the discussion of tuberculosis. Emaciation often accompanies chronic, wasting diseases such as TB and cancer. Dehydration is also characteristic of these conditions, as it is with acute, febrile, infections such as pneumonia. Febrile diseases also predispose to rapid blood coagulation, and the high bacterial activity associated with these diseases can result in more rapid decomposition than normal.

Edema, especially hydrothorax, is also a common condition associated with respiratory infections. fluid collecting in the thoracic area not only has the effect of diluting primary solutions of embalming chemicals, but its mere presence in significant amounts can put pressure on surrounding vessels and impede the normal flow of chemicals through the vascular system.

Pulmonary infections such as pneumonia, with their accompanying exudates, predispose to poor oxygenation of the blood moving through the lungs. Consequently, **cyanosis,** or a bluish discoloration of the tissues is likely to result, and can persist after death as a discoloration to be dealt with by the embalmer.

All of these post-mortem conditions require that the embalming operator select the best possible combination of embalming chemicals and techniques which will help to overcome such conditions as a high bacterial count, blood coagulation, edema, and discolorations.

Chapter Ten
DISEASES OF THE URINARY SYSTEM

Anatomy Review

The urinary system is important for its function of removing waste products from the body. When cellular metabolism occurs throughout the body, various chemical waste products result and are picked up by the bloodstream. These waste products need to be filtered out of the blood and eliminated before they build up to toxic levels. This filtering process is accomplished by the kidneys, which are also important for their role in maintaining proper water, electrolyte, and acid-base balance in the body.

The nephron is the basic structural and functional unit of kidney tissue, which in turn consists of a renal corpuscle and a renal tubule. The renal corpuscle is a capsule containing a specialized group of blood capillaries called a glomerulus, through which water and waste products are filtered out of the blood. This filtered solution then enters the renal tubule, where most of the water, plus needed nutrients and other elements are reabsorbed through the walls of the tubules back into the bloodstream. The water and waste products which are left over is called urine, and is secreted by the many renal tubules into the kidney pelvis. The kidney pelvis then passes urine into the ureter, which is the tube carrying urine to the urinary bladder. When a sufficient quantity of urine accumulates in the bladder, it is expelled from the body through the urethra, or the exit tube from the bladder.

Diseases of the Kidney

Nephritis, or inflammation of the kidney, may take many forms. **Glomerulonephritis** refers to inflammation of the glomeruli, which are the filtering capillaries in the kidney. Glomerulonephritis is usually an allergic or autoimmune type of disease, similar to rheumatic fever. It is characterized by damage to the walls of the glomeruli as a result of antigen-antibody reactions which occur following a previous streptococcal infection. As a result of the damage done to the glomeruli, substances such as blood cells and serum albumin, a plasma protein, often show up in the urine. Blood in the urine is called **hematuria,** and albumin in the urine is referred to as **albuminuria.**

Glomerulonephritis may be either acute or chronic in nature. Chronic glomerulonephritis is often accompanied by hypertension. In fact, hypertension often leads to kidney disease, but conversely, kidney disease may also lead to hypertension. When a diseased kidney is not functioning properly, this results in excess water and salts building up in the bloodstream, which has the effect of raising blood pressure.

Other parts of the kidney may also be affected by disease. When the arteries and arterioles of the kidney become hardened and sclerotic, it is referred to as **nephrosclerosis.** Inflammation of the kidney pelvis, which is the expanded upper part of the ureter, is referred to as **pyelitis,** and inflammation of the pelvis and the kidney itself is called **pyelonephritis.** These common kidney infections are usually caused by pyogenic bacteria which may reach the kidney either via the bloodstream or by migrating up from the lower part of the urinary tract. *(See Fig. 35)*

63

Various diseases of the kidney, including forms of nephritis, result in the inability of the kidney to properly filter waste products out of the bloodstream. These waste products, such as urea and uric acid, result from normal, everyday cellular metabolism, and it is the job of the kidney to remove them from the body. If a diseased kidney cannot filter waste products out of the blood, the condition called **uremia** results. This condition can be serious, and even fatal, if the cause of the toxic build-up is not eliminated.

Kidney failure, with associated changes in the normal volume of urine output, may occur in various degrees, and may be either acute or chronic. Complete suppression of urine output, indicating total kidney failure, is referred to as **anuria** (an = none, uria = urine), while **oliguria** (olig = little) indicates less than the normal amount of urine.

The condition called **polyuria** (poly=much) refers to the passage of excess quantities of urine, and although it sometimes accompanies chronic nephritis, it is often an indication of problems elsewhere in the body. **Diabetes insipidus** is actually a disease of the posterior part of the pituitary gland, which is responsible for secreting anti-diuretic hormone. This hormone regulates urine output by preventing the kidney from passing too much water out through the urinary system. When this hormone is not properly produced, excess urine is generated, and polyuria results. This can lead to a rapid and serious dehydration of the body if not corrected.

Also, polyuria often accompanies **diabetes mellitus**, or the more common "sugar diabetes". **Glycosuria,** or excess sugar in the urine, is also commonly associated with diabetes mellitus. In this form of diabetes, the pancreas is not producing insulin which is necessary for the proper metabolism of carbohydrates, and sugars tend to build up in the bloodstream and spill over into the urinary system. While neither form of diabetes is considered a disease of the kidneys, they are mentioned here because they result in conditions which are observed through the functioning of the urinary system.

As was mentioned earlier, **hematuria** refers to blood in the urine, and often accompanies glomerulonephritis, kidney infections, tumors, and other urinary system diseases. However, occasionally only hemoglobin is present in the urine, not whole blood. This would be called **hemoglobinuria,** and is more likely to accompany disease of the blood, such as hemolytic anemias, where red cells are being abnormally destroyed. As a result of red cell destruction, excess hemoglobin can pass through the urinary system and show up in the urine.

The kidneys are also often affected by genetic or developmental abnormalities, such as **hypoplasia,** meaning underdevelopment of a body part, and **polycystic kidney disease**. In this disease, the kidneys develop numerous cysts, which often become enlarged and compress surrounding tissue, and are prone to infection. This cyst formation adversely affects normal kidney function, and may lead to uremia and kidney failure. *(See Fig. 36)*

Other Urinary System Diseases

Hydronephrosis is a condition which is characterized by a build-up of urine in the kidney pelvis, causing a dilation of the pelvis and even compression of kidney tissue. The problem usually occurs as a result of a blockage somewhere along the urinary tract. Blockages are often caused by such things as tumors, stricture from scar tissue, and kidney stones. *(See Fig. 37 and Fig. 38)*

The formation of kidney stones is called **nephrolithiasis.** The stones themselves are called **nephroliths,** or **renal calculi**. They commonly form in the kidney pelvis, and may block the ureters, or if they are small enough, pass into the bladder, continue to grow, and eventually block the urethra. Stones also predispose to irritation and infection of the lining of the urinary tract. They often form when mineral salts present in the urine precipitate out of solution. Their formation is sometimes associated with kidney inflammation, certain dietary problems, and hyperparathyroidism.

Other inflammations of the urinary tract are identified based on their anatomical location. **Ureteritis** is inflammation of the ureters, **cystitis** is inflammation of the urinary bladder, and **urethritis** is inflammation of the urethra. Many urinary tract infections are caused by pyogenic bacteria, resulting in pus formation, and the condition of having pus in the urine is referred to as **pyuria.** Organisms which commonly cause infection of the urinary tract include *Neisseria gonorrhea, Chlamydia trachomatis, Escherichia coli, Proteus species, Pseudomonas species,* and *Treponema pallidum.*

Carcinomas are common malignant tumors which occur in the urinary system. The bladder is regularly affected by a variety referred to as transitional cell carcinomas. The kidney is often affected by tumors as well, with one common type, generally affecting adults, referred to as renal cell carcinoma. Wilm's tumor is the name given to a malignant, rapid growing kidney tumor often seen in young children. These neoplasms are often of the mixed variety, with epithelial, muscle, and connective tissues involved in the same tumor.

Embalming Considerations

Uremia caused by kidney failure can have an adverse effect on the embalming operation. Urea, and other toxic waste products in the blood, have the effect of altering tissue proteins so that the ability of formaldehyde to coagulate these proteins is diminished. This result, plus the neutralizing effect of the waste products themselves on formaldehyde, leads to an increased formaldehyde demand in order to properly firm and preserve the tissues of the body.

In addition to the presence of metabolic waste products in the body, kidney disease also can result in **edema,** as excess water is not properly removed from the body by the kidneys, increasing secondary dilution of the embalming fluid. The toxic waste products which have built up have the further effect of causing vascular damage, increased capillary permeability, and consequently a greater likelihood for edema to occur.

As a result of the uremia which occurs, a **strong odor** of urine in the tissues may be present. This odor problem is yet another concern for the embalmer, which can be greatly improved with the proper use of sufficient quantities of embalming chemicals.

In general, it can be said that bodies which are affected by kidney disease, with its resulting uremia, edema, and odor problems, will require a stronger than normal arterial solution in order to overcome these difficulties. Of course, each case should be thoroughly evaluated on a case by case basis, with individual case differences determining the best procedures to be employed.

Chapter Eleven

DISEASES OF THE NERVOUS SYSTEM

Anatomy Review

The nervous system is the body's highly complex system for controlling various bodily functions. It can be thought of as a communications network, with information coming into the main part of the system from all over the body, having it processed, and a resulting flow of instructions and commands traveling in the opposite direction to the body parts. In the nervous system, this flow of information occurs in the form of electrical impulses which travel over highly specialized nerve cells to and from the brain and spinal cord.

Nerve cells, or neurons, are body cells specialized for the purpose of transmitting stimuli they receive either toward the central nervous system, or away from the central nervous system. If a neuron is transmitting a stimulus such as one from heat, cold, or touch toward the central nervous system, it is called a sensory neuron. If the neurons's job is to transmit a stimulus such as a command for muscular movement, or one for the release of digestive enzymes by a gland, away from the central nervous system, it is called a motor neuron.

The nervous system can be divided into two main parts, referred to as the central nervous system, which includes the brain and spinal cord, and the peripheral nervous system, which includes all of the nerves through which the brain and spinal cord communicate with the various body parts.

Three main subdivisions of the brain include the cerebrum, the cerebellum, and the brain stem. The brain stem is continuous with the spinal cord which is encased within the vertebrae making up the spinal column. The brain gives off twelve pairs of cranial nerves and the spinal cord gives off thirty-one pairs of spinal nerves. These cranial and spinal nerves are the pathways which allow the brain and spinal cord to communicate with all parts of the body.

The brain and spinal cord are covered over by three layers of protective membranes called the meninges. They are identified, from outer to inner, as the dura mater, the arachnoid mater, and the pia mater.

Also contained within the brain are four cavities called ventricles, which are involved in secreting cerebrospinal fluid derived from blood plasma. This fluid flows out of the ventricles and surrounds the brain and spinal cord in the sub-arachnoid space.

Traumatic Diseases

Trauma to the head is a common occurrence, and cerebral hemorrhages are often categorized based on where the hemorrhage occurs in relation to the meninges. Hemorrhage which occurs outside of the dura, between the dura and the cranial bones, is called **extra-dural,** or sometimes **epidural,** hemorrhage. If the hemorrhage occurs beneath the dura, between it and the arachnoid, it is referred to as a **sub-dural** hemorrhage. Hemorrhages underneath the arachnoid, between it and the pia, are identified as **sub-arachnoid** hemorrhages. These hemorrhages may result from various forms of injury to the head, or they may follow the rupture of a weakened or diseased blood vessel in the brain. *(See Fig. 39)*

The term **contusion** is often used to describe an injury to the brain where the skin has not been broken at the site of the injury. In other words, a bruising of the brain, accompanied by swelling and pain. If bone is broken in an injury, it would be referred to as a **fracture,** and the brain itself could even be subject to tearing or **laceration** if the injury is serious enough.

Concussion is a term which describes the results of receiving a blow to the head without actually suffering other serious lesions such as a fracture, laceration, or hemorrhage. It may simply result in a temporary grogginess, or may be more serious, with widespread loss of cerebral control and depressed vital signs.

Infectious Diseases

Many infectious diseases caused by bacteria and viruses have significant effects upon nervous tissue in the body. Damage done may be a direct result of the organism itself affecting the tissue, or as a result of products such as bacterial toxins which do the ultimate damage. Infectious diseases affecting the nervous system are often referred to as **neurotropic** diseases.

Encephalitis is a general term referring to inflammation of the brain. One of the most common forms of the disease is viral encephalitis, which is an infection often transmitted to humans via the bites of infected mosquitoes. The virus responsible for this infection commonly resides in wild birds and some mammals such as horses. Mosquitoes then serve as the vectors by transmitting the virus from these animals to humans. One form of the disease is referred to as "equine encephalitis", indicating horses as the normal reservoir for the infection.

Besides being a viral infection, encephalitis may also be a complication of other infectious diseases such as malaria, influenza, measles, and typhus fever. If the spinal cord is also involved in the infection, as it often is, it may be referred to as encephalomyelitis.

Meningitis indicates an inflammation of the meninges surrounding the brain and spinal cord. The disease may take many forms and is caused by numerous organisms, including viruses and various bacteria. Common bacteria causing meningitis include *Hemophilus influenzae, Streptococcus pneumoniae (pneumococcus)* and *Neisseria meningitidis (meningococcus).* Meningitis caused by the meningococcus is often referred to as epidemic meningitis, and is one of the most serious forms of the disease. It is commonly transmitted from person to person through the respiratory tract via droplet spray or direct contact with respiratory discharges. Organisms causing meningitis usually reach the meninges either via the blood or lymph stream from other areas in the body, or as extensions of local infections such as otitis media and mastoiditis.

Meningitis is characterized by fever, chills, severe headache, and a stiff, painful neck. It may progress to involve nausea, vomiting, and convulsions. If not properly treated, the disease can result in serious brain damage and even death. *(See Fig. 40)*

Myelitis refers to inflammation of the spinal cord, and it may result from infection, or as an after effect of injury to the spinal cord. **Poliomyelitis** is an important form of myelitis, and indicates an inflammation of the gray matter in the cord. Although its name designates localization in the spinal cord, it often involves brain matter as well. This disease is a viral infection primarily affecting motor neurons in the central nervous system, which may result in serious nerve damage and paralysis of muscles controlled by these nerves.

Poliomyelitis used to be a severe, crippling disease, but its incidence in the United States has been nearly eradicated over the last several decades due to the discovery of the Salk and Sabin vaccines, which are routinely given to young children as a preventative measure.

The term **neuritis** refers to inflammation of a nerve or nerves. It may result from a number of causes, such as direct infection of the nerves, or as a complication of other infections such as tuberculosis, tetanus, or measles. Neuritis can also result from mechanical factors such as trauma or contusion. Toxins and poisons of various types may also lead to inflammation of a nerve.

Rabies is an infection which tends to affect the nervous system, and is often fatal if contracted and untreated. It is common to many forms of animals, including raccoons, foxes, skunks, bats, and dogs. The disease is most often transmitted to humans through infected saliva obtained from animal bites.

Circulatory Disorders

We have previously mentioned several forms of cerebral hemorrhage, based on the location of the hemorrhage in reference to the meninges. In addition to these forms of hemorrhage, special note should be made of circulatory interruption occurring in the brain which falls under the general heading of **stroke, apoplexy,** or **cerebrovascular accident (CVA).**

A stroke can be described as damage to the brain as a result of circulatory interruption. Brain tissue is extremely sensitive to the loss of oxygen, and when circulation is interrupted, the effects can range from mild to fatal, depending on the size and location of the artery involved. Mild strokes often result in partial, and only temporary, loss of such functions as sight, speech, motion, and sensation. More severe strokes result in permanent loss of these functions, and may even prove fatal within a short time after occurring. The most common causes of stroke include thrombosis, embolism, and hemorrhage.

A **transient ischemic attack** (TIA) is a temporary interference with the blood supply to a part of the brain. Unlike a stroke, no permanent damage usually occurs. An attack may be characterized by dizziness, fuzzy vision in one eye, or a numbness or loss of sensation on one side of the body. TIA's may last for only a few moments, or up to several hours.

Other Nervous System Diseases

Hydrocephalus, or water on the brain, is a condition which results when there is a blockage to the normal outflow of cerebrospinal fluid. This fluid is secreted by special capillaries within the ventricles of the brain, and normally exits the ventricles to flow around the brain and spinal cord in the sub-arachnoid space. When there is a lesion of some sort which does not allow the cerebrospinal fluid to exit from the ventricles, it continues to build up and compresses the surrounding brain tissue against the cranial bones. The resulting damage to the nervous system can be serious enough to cause extensive loss of cerebral function and vital life processes. Severe cases of the disease either result in stillbirths, or a brief life span of only days or weeks.

Although hydrocephalus may be either congenital or acquired, the most striking examples of the disease occur in young babies. Due to the fact that ossification of the cranial bones has not yet occurred, a great distention and enlargement of the cranium can be observed. When it occurs in adults, the cranial enlargement is not seen, because hardening of the bones has already taken place. Acquired hydrocephalus is often seen when post-inflammatory adhesions or scarring occurs, or with some cases of meningitis. Also, the growth of tumors may result in a blockage to the normal flow of cerebrospinal fluid.

Epilepsy is a condition which results from some form of interference with normal electrical activity in the brain. Many cases of epilepsy are of unknown cause, but others have been associated with brain injury, trauma at birth, or tumors.

The most prominent feature of epilepsy is the convulsions which tend to occur. In **grand mal** epilepsy, which is the more serious form of the disease, the patient may experience strong convulsions, make peculiar sounds, bite the tongue, and show excess salivation. The seizures of epilepsy vary considerably in the length of duration and frequency of occurrence. After an attack, patients are usually somewhat groggy, and not fully aware of what has occurred.

A milder form of epilepsy, **petite mal**, may be characterized by only dizziness and a brief loss of consciousness. This form of the disease is more common in children, and may disappear completely by early adulthood.

Multiple sclerosis is a chronic, degenerative disease affecting the nervous system. It usually affects young adults from about 20-40 years of age. Although the real cause of the disease remains unknown, many theories have been put forth, including a genetic anomaly, bacterial and viral involvement, and immune reactions against viral infections.

Multiple sclerosis is characterized by a destruction of the myelin sheaths, or outer coverings around nerve fibers. As a result of this tissue destruction, both motor and sensory nerve impulses tend to become impaired. The patient may experience such conditions as muscular weakness and incoordination, tremors, paralysis, vision problems, and abnormal, rapid eyeball movements.

The name of the disease is derived from the fact that the damaged nervous tissue tends to become replaced with multiple sites of hardened, or sclerotic plaques, such as those which affect the vascular system in arteriosclerosis.

Another chronic, degenerative disease of the nervous system is **Parkinson's disease.** It tends to develop later in life, and can be very debilitating, with no real cure available. The disease, sometimes referred to as "shaking palsy", is characterized by slow spreading tremors, especially in the hands and fingers, muscular rigidity, and a peculiar gait. The person tends to have an expressionless face with slow and deliberate speech. The posture of a Parkinson's patient is stooped forward, with the head flexed to the chest, wrists flexed, and the knees bent. Walking occurs in short, rapid steps, often resulting in the loss of balance and falling.

Recovery from Parkinson's rarely occurs, and only drug treatment for some of the muscular rigidity and tremors is helpful in making the patient more comfortable.

Cerebral palsy is a nervous system disorder affecting young children, but unlike diseases such as multiple sclerosis and Parkinson's, it is not a progressive type of condition. Usually as a result of some sort of brain damage either before birth or shortly thereafter, a child is affected with motor disorders and possibly some mental retardation. The child tends to walk on the toes, with the knees bent and pointed inward. Mild cases of the condition respond well if early therapy is available, but more severe cases may show retardation, permanent paralysis, and even convulsions.

Creutzfeldt-Jakob disease is a somewhat rare yet deadly disease which causes a slow degeneration of the central nervous system, resulting in a gradual mental deterioration called dementia. It was originally thought to be caused by a conventional virus, but scientists now believe that a small, protein particle called a prion is responsible for this disease.

Creutzfeldt-Jakob, and other so called "slow virus" infections, may remain dormant in the body for extended periods of time, even years, before causing any signs of illness. Although the infection may lie dormant for many years, once symptoms develop, it usually proves fatal within about a year.

This disease does not appear to be a contagious type of infection, and the only likelihood of contracting it is through a penetrating injury by something contaminated with the infectious agent. Therefore, as with other infectious diseases, the most important consideration in the preparation room is careful technique and avoidance of self-inflicted injuries.

Alzheimer's disease is a nervous system disorder characterized by loss of memory, mood changes, and other mental disturbances. It is not believed to be caused by conventional infectious agents such as bacteria and viruses, and the real cause of the disease remains a mystery.

Alzheimer's is characterized by destruction of neurons in the cortex of the brain, with a corresponding deposition of plaques upon the nerve fibers. It gradually causes loss of mental faculties over many years, and may ultimately result in near total loss of all motor and intellectual abilities.

Embalming Considerations

Infectious diseases of the nervous system should be treated as any other infectious disease, with care being given to assuring adequate disinfection through all phases of the embalming operation. Of special concern should be the treatment of the cranial cavity. Rapid decomposition of the brain due to a high bacterial count can predispose to distention of the eyeballs and brain purge. Care should be taken to aspirate the cranial cavity, with injection of an appropriate amount of cavity fluid into the cavity, in order to counter these difficulties.

Hemorrhages, such as petechiae, are also common complications of infections such as meningitis, and may be present as post-mortem conditions. Organisms causing meningitis often spread from the nasopharynx, into the bloodstream, before reaching the nervous system. In some cases of meningococcemia, the resulting septicemia is so severe that death may result from adrenal and other hemorrhages before the nervous system is greatly involved.

Another post-mortem condition which may present itself in certain nervous system diseases is atrophy of body organs or parts. When chronic, degenerative diseases of the nervous system adversely affect the ability of the brain and spinal cord to communicate with body organs, these organs tend to atrophy as a result of this lost nervous stimulation. This may present the embalmer with the need to treat body parts which are abnormal in size or shape as a result of this atrophy.

Chapter Twelve

DISEASES OF THE REPRODUCTIVE SYSTEM

The Male Reproductive System

Anatomy Review

The male reproductive system is responsible for producing spermatozoa, the male sex cells, which are introduced into the reproductive tract of the female in order to fertilize an egg.

The male sexual organs, or gonads, are referred to as the testes. They are contained within the scrotum, which is a sac-like structure suspended from the lower, anterior pelvic region. Contained within the testes are structures called seminiferous tubules where the spermatozoa are produced. The spermatozoa then travel from the testes into the spermatic duct, and eventually leave the body through the urethra. The spermatic duct consists of three main sections, identified as the epididymis, the vas deferens, and the ejaculatory duct.

Accessory glands which provide secretions to aid in the movement and nurturing of spermatozoa include the seminal vesicles, the bulbourethral glands, and the prostate gland.

The penis is an organ which consists of several layers of erectile tissue, and contains the terminal portions of the urethra, through which spermatozoa are introduced into the female reproductive tract.

In addition to spermatozoa, the testes also produce testosterone, which is the sex hormone involved in development of male sexual characteristics.

Inflammatory Diseases

Inflammation of the testes is referred to as orchitis. It is most often a complication of other infectious diseases, especially mumps. If the infection is serious enough, it may result in scarring, atrophy of the testes, and even sterility.

Epididymitis is inflammation of the epididymis, the highly twisted and tortuous initial section of the spermatic duct. It generally results from an initial infection of gonococcal urethritis. It is usually treatable with antibiotics, but severe cases, especially if they are bi-lateral, may lead to scarring of the epididymis, disallowing the passage of sperm and resulting in sterility.

Prostatitis, or inflammation of the prostate gland, is another infection which is often secondary to cases of urethritis. Organisms such as *Neisseria gonorrhea* and *Escherichia coli* account for many cases of the disease. It is characterized by pain, swelling, possible pus formation, and may lead to compression of the urethra, resulting in interference with the passage of urine.

Many inflammations of the reproductive tract are sexually transmitted diseases. Four of the most common sexually transmitted diseases include gonorrhea, syphilis, non-specific urethritis, and genital herpes.

Gonorrhea is an infection of the reproductive tract caused by *Neisseria gonorrhea*. It is characterized by suppuration, and may lead to sterility if not properly treated.

Syphilis is an infection caused by the spirochete *Treponema pallidum*. It is a highly invasive infection, which is generally characterized by three stages of development, referred to as the primary, secondary, and tertiary stages.

Primary syphilis is normally accompanied by an ulceration called a hard **chancre**. This genital sore usually appears several weeks after initial contact, and may persist for four to six weeks, after which it heals.

The signs of secondary syphilis generally begin to occur in several additional weeks, and may persist for months and even years. Two of the signs associated with secondary syphilis are a generalized red **skin rash**, and small ulcerations on the mucous membranes, especially in the mouth, called **mucous patches**. By the time these indications of secondary syphilis present themselves, it is evidence that this invasive organism has spread throughout the body to cause its damage.

Tertiary syphilis, which may take years to develop, is characterized by areas of necrotic tissue called **gumma**. These lesions develop over time as a result of the persistent inflammatory responses in the body to the presence of the spirochete causing the disease. Although nearly any area of the body may be affected, the cardiovascular and nervous systems seem to be most commonly diseased.

Neurosyphilis may lead to damage to the brain, resulting in a mental deterioration and paralysis called general **paresis** (Gr. = weakness). When damage to the spinal cord occurs, it usually causes a degeneration of the posterior part of the cord, hence the designation **tabes dorsalis** (L. tabes = a wasting) is given to this form of the disease. Neurosyphilis may also affect the meninges, resulting in syphilitic **meningitis**.

In the cardiovascular system, syphilis has a tendency to affect the arteries, especially the aorta, causing inflammation and **aneurysms**. It also damages the aortic valve, causing aortic insufficiency.

Another sexually transmitted disease, non-specific urethritis, is an infection most often caused by a chlamydia organism. NSU is one of the most common and widespread of the sexually transmitted diseases.

Genital herpes, caused by the Herpes simplex II virus, is a sexually transmitted disease characterized by painful, itchy ulcerations or blisters which tend to occur on the genitals and surrounding areas. There is no cure for genital herpes, and it tends to be a recurrent disease, with healing of the lesions occurring after an active period. However, the virus remains dormant in the body, and may reactivate itself at various times, often as a result of stress or other periods of low resistance.

A build-up of edematous fluid in the scrotum, surrounding the testes, is called **hydrocele**. It may complicate inflammations such as orchitis or epididymitis, or it may result from improper closure of the opening between the peritoneal cavity and the scrotum. If the latter occurs, peritoneal fluid may collect in the scrotum causing swelling and pressure on the testes.

Other Male Reproductive Diseases

Although we have previously mentioned enlargement of the prostate in reference to inflammation, a fairly common condition called benign prostatic hyperplasia, often affects men over fifty years of age. This is not an inflammatory condition, nor necessarily a pre-cancerous one, but is often associated with a hormone imbalance in later years. The main problem caused by this prostatic enlargement is interference with the passage of urine. This in turn can result in hypertrophy of the bladder, ureters, and kidney pelvis. This collection of urine then predisposes to infections of the urinary tract.

In the developmental process, before birth the male testes are situated in the pelvic cavity, and normally descend into the scrotum shortly before birth. If this does not occur, the condition is referred to as **cryptorchism** (cryptorchidism).

In order for sperm to properly develop, the testes need to be located within the scrotum, and not in the pelvic cavity where the temperature is slightly higher. Failure of the testes to descend into the scrotum can lead to sterility. Drug therapy, and possibly surgery, are often successful in correcting the condition of cryptorchism.

Carcinomas affecting the male reproductive tract are most common in the prostate gland and testes. Prostatic carcinoma is fairly common in older men, and the prognosis for the disease is not good if it has become established, as it tends to metastasize quite rapidly to other parts of the body, especially the bones and lymph nodes.

Testicular tumors are usually malignant, but fortunately they are much less common than prostatic cancer. Unlike tumors of the prostate, these tumors tend to affect younger men in their 20's, 30's, and 40's.

The Female Reproductive System

Anatomy Review

The female reproductive system is responsible for the production of the ovum, or egg, which is fertilized by the male spermatozoa, and the ensuing period of growth and development results in the birth of a new child.

Ova are produced in the female ovary, and are expelled from the ovary in a process called ovulation. The ovum enters the fallopian tube, which is a passageway between the ovary and the uterus. Fertilization normally occurs in the fallopian tube, after which the fertilized ovum eventually enters the uterus, attaches itself to the inner lining of the uterus, and develops there over the nine month period of gestation.

The main parts of the uterus include the fundus, which is the upper dome-shaped part, the body, which is the main central portion, and the cervix, which is the inferior constricted segment. The uterus consists mainly of a thick muscular layer called the myometrium. Lining the inside of the myometrium is the endometrium, and covering over the outside of this muscular layer is the perimetrium.

The vagina is a canal-like passageway which extends from the bottom of the cervix to the outer genital area. The term vestibule is used to identify the entranceway into the vagina from the outside.

The external genitals include the labia minora and the labia majora, the clitoris, and the mons pubis.

Inflammatory Diseases

As with other body areas, inflammation involving the female reproductive organs are identified based on the specific organ affected. **Oophoritis** refers to inflammation of the ovaries, **salpingitis** is inflammation of the fallopian tubes, and **metritis**, or **uteritis**, is inflammation of the uterus. One of the more common forms of metritis is **endometritis**, which indicates inflammation of the inner lining of the uterus. If the lining of the cervix is inflamed, it is referred to as **endocervicitis**. **Vaginitis** involves inflammation of the vagina, and **mastitis** is inflammation of the mammary glands, or breasts. In addition, abscess formation is quite common in the ovaries and fallopian tubes. *(See Fig. 41)*

Numerous organisms can lead to these inflammations of the reproductive tract, including the gonococcus, staphylococcus, chlamydia, and streptococcus organisms. One danger which may occur as a result of inflammation of the fallopian tubes is sterility, particularly if the disease is bi-lateral and is not properly treated with antibiotics. Scar tissues can form which effectively closes off the tube, disallowing the passage of an ovum, and consequently preventing a normal pregnancy.

A common cause of vaginitis is a yeast infection caused by the fungus *Candida albicans*. This often occurs as a complication of antibiotic therapy for another bodily infection, which may have the effect of destroying normal flora present in the vaginal area, and allowing a greater foothold for the offending fungal organism.

Other common infections of the female reproductive tract include puerperal sepsis and toxic shock syndrome. Puerperal sepsis is an infection of the reproductive tract following childbirth, usually streptococcal in origin. During this time period the body is particularly susceptible to infection due to ruptured vessels and the exposed nature of the endometrium following delivery.

Toxic shock syndrome is a staphylococcal infection of the reproductive tract, often associated with prolonged tampon usage, which can provide an en-vironment suitable for bacterial growth and toxin production.

Syphilis and herpes infections, previously discussed in the section on the male reproductive system, also may affect the female reproductive tract.

Other Diseases of the Female Reproductive Tract

Occasionally a condition occurs in pregnant women, normally during the third trimester, which is sometimes referred to as toxemia of pregnancy, although no real toxins are found in the body. The condition is usually characterized by edema of the extremities and the face area, high blood pressure, and a high albuminuria, or the presence of serum albumin in the urine. The cause of the disease is unknown, and if not treated it can lead to the condition called **eclampsia**, which is characterized by convulsions, coma, and even death. It is thought by many experts that pre-existing high blood pressure and glomerulonephritis predispose to the development of eclampsia.

Fertilization of an ovum by a spermatozoa normally occurs in the fallopian tube. Occasionally this fertilized ovum is not able to pass out of the tube and attach itself to the endometrium of the uterus. This interference with passage of the egg may be associated with various conditions such as tumors, adhesions, or previous cases of salpingitis. When a **tubal pregnancy** of this sort occurs, an embryo may attempt to develop in the tube, but is unable to sustain long-term growth at this location, and will likely lead to either rupture of the tube or tubal abortion. *(See Fig. 42 and 43)*

Less common than a tubal pregnancy is an **abdominal pregnancy**, where a fertilized ovum attempts to develop in the abdominal cavity. It is possible that fertilization occurred in this abnormal location, and the egg was never able to make it into the fallopian tube. Both of these forms of pregnancy are examples of pregnancy occurring outside of the uterus, and are therefore referred to as extrauterine, or ectopic, pregnancies.

Endometriosis is a condition where endometrial tissue, normally found lining the uterus, is located elsewhere in the pelvic or abdominal area. Areas of this tissue may be found on the fallopian tubes, ovaries, peritoneum, intestines, etc. When located in these unusual places, endometrial tissue can only create problems, and usually leads to pain, swelling, and bleeding at the site. It is not totally clear how this tissue comes to be located in these areas, but theories include such things as backward flow of endometrial tissue through the fallopian tubes during menstruation, blood or lymph stream spread of endometrial cells, and implantation of these cells in abnormal areas during surgery.

Ovarian cysts are another common condition affecting the female reproductive tract. One form of ovarian cyst, called a **dermoid cyst**, is a benign neoplasm containing a rather greasy material secreted by sebaceous glands formed in the walls of the cyst. It may also contain other bodily tissues not normally found in this area, such as hair, skin, thyroid tissue, and even teeth.

Tumors of various types also affect the female organs of reproduction. One of the more common types of ovarian tumors develops from the surface epithelium of the ovary, and is referred to as a cystadenoma, or cystadenocarcinoma if malignant. This tumor is so called due to the excessive secretion of fluid by glandular epithelium which tends to form cysts in the ovary.

Uterine cancer is also quite common, with the cervix area being the most often affected part of the uterus. Cervical cancers, generally squamous cell carcinomas of the endometrium, are one of the most common forms of malignancy affecting women world-wide. *(See Fig. 44)*

Leiomyomas of the uterus, sometimes referred to a fibroid tumors, are very common benign tumors which develop from the smooth muscle fibers in the walls of the uterus. They may grow to fill the entire uterine cavity if not removed. *(See Fig. 45)*

Along with cervical cancer, carcinoma of the breast is one of the most common forms of cancer in women, and it is responsible for thousands of deaths each year in this country (upwards of 40,000 per year by some estimates). This form of cancer tends to spread, infiltrating the surrounding muscles and skin. It also spreads quite rapidly through the blood and lymphatic vessels in the chest area, often requiring removal of these surrounding tissues and lymph nodes when surgery is deemed necessary. Surgical removal of a breast is referred to as **mastectomy**.

Self examination for the early detection of lumps in the breast is seen as an important measure in discovering and controlling the development of breast cancer.

Embalming Considerations

Diseases of the reproductive tract, both male and female, do not present a lot of unusual embalming problems. Certainly the various infectious diseases should be given the same consideration as any other infectious disease, with care taken to use an embalming solution of sufficient strength to provide adequate disinfection. In cases where external lesions are present, such as those of genital herpes, surface treatment of the affected area with disinfectant compresses or hypodermic injection may be necessary.

As with infectious diseases in general, those affecting the reproductive tracts can predispose to **rapid blood coagulation**, especially if they become systemic in nature. **Ascites** may also be a problem is some cases of infection or tumor growth in the pelvic area.

One condition of particular concern is **hydrocele**, or a build-up of edematous fluid in the scrotum. Hydrocele can present a case of great distention of the scrotal area, requiring the embalmer to pay particular attention to this condition. In an effort to reduce this distention, the scrotum should be treated separately, preferably by aspiration with an infant trocar, then by injecting several ounces of an astringent embalming chemical, such as cavity fluid, into the scrotum. This will help reduce the swelling and neutralize the likelihood of more rapid decomposition due to an area of untreated edema.

Chapter Thirteen

DISEASES OF THE BONES AND JOINTS

Anatomy Review

There are 206 classified bones in the human skeleton, 80 of which are in the axial skeleton and 126 make up the appendicular skeleton. The axial skeleton includes the skull, spine, rib cage, sternum, and hyoid bone. The appendicular skeleton includes the upper extremities and the pectoral girdle, and the lower extremities plus the pelvic girdle.

Bones serve some important functions, including protection of interior organs, providing body rigidity, serving as points for muscle attachments, and acting as a warehouse or storage area for various minerals the body needs. In addition, the bones of the body are important for their function of producing blood cells, which is a constant, day to day activity, as blood cells routinely wear out and need to be replaced.

Bones are developed from connective tissue, and come in a variety of shapes. They may be flat, irregular, short, or long. Whatever their shape, they all contain a dense, outer layer called compact bone, and a more spongy, inner layer called cancellous bone. The long bones also possess an inner cavity referred to as the medullary canal.

Covering over the outer surface of a bone is a tough layer of fibrous connective tissue referred to as the periosteum. The periosteum contains many blood vessels and specialized cells capable of forming new bone tissue, and also serves as the attachment point for tendons, which function to attach the muscles of the body to the bones.

The point of union of two bones is called an articulation, or joint. Joints are often classified based on the amount of movement which occurs at the site. An immovable articulation, such as the cranial sutures, is called a synarthrosis, a slightly movable articulation, such as the pubic symphysis, is called an amphiarthrosis, and a freely movable articulation, such as the knee joint, is referred to as a diarthrosis.

Ligaments are tough bands of connective tissue which attach bones to each other. In addition to ligaments, a diarthrosis contains a capsule which encloses the entire joint. This capsule is lined with a lubricating layer of tissue called a synovial membrane, which secretes synovial fluid.

Cartilage is a flexible, elastic form of connective tissue, which serves to cushion the ends of articulating bones. It is also found in areas where shape or form is important, but the rigidity of bone is not necessary, such as in the nose, ears, and larynx.

Inflammatory Diseases of Bone

Osteitis refers to inflammation of a bone, and it may take many forms. One of the more common types is called osteitis fibrosa cystica, which is characterized by the formation of cysts and fibrous nodules within bones. This is thought to be a result of a hormone imbalance involving the parathyroid gland, which is involved in regulation of blood calcium levels. Hyperparathyroidism can lead to decalcification of the bones, which leads to a loss of bone density and cyst formation.

Paget's disease, or osteitis deformans, is a chronic inflammation of bones resulting in thickening and deformation. The cause in unknown, and generally affects the elderly. Bone which has undergone these changes is also predisposed to malignant developments, often with the formation of osteosarcomas.

Bone tissue may also be inflamed by the invasion of microorganisms, such as the bacillus causing tuberculosis, or the spirochete *Treponema pallidum*, which is the causative agent for syphilis.

Osteomyelitis is a condition where the bone marrow, and possibly the bone as well, is inflamed. It may result from organisms entering the bone as an after effect of trauma, such as with various fractures, or it may be a focal infection which has spread to the bones from other areas in the body via the blood or lymph streams. One common example of this happening is mastoiditis, or inflammation of the mastoid portion of the temporal bone, which may occur as an extension of chronic otitis media.

Arthritis, referring to inflammation of a joint, is an extremely common condition, and it may occur in literally dozens of forms. Arthritis may result from such things as trauma, tumors, degenerative conditions accompanying old age, allergic reactions, or from infectious agents like bacteria, fungi, and viruses. Arthritis may also be either acute or chronic in nature.

Rheumatoid arthritis is one common form of chronic arthritis, affecting mainly women and beginning in the younger years from approximately 20-40 years of age. It generally begins as an inflammation of the synovial membrane lining the joint capsule, and there tends to be a bi-lateral involvement of the hand and wrist joints in the beginning. Often developing in other areas of the body as time passes.

Rheumatoid arthritis is often accompanied by general systemic reactions such as fever, weight loss, and anemia. In the later stages of the disease, a joint may be totally destroyed, and the articular surfaces fuse together, causing a permanent crippling. The disease is also characterized by the formation of hard, subcutaneous nodules which form in the vicinity of the joints, particularly on the arms near the elbow area.

The cause of rheumatoid arthritis is somewhat obscure, but many experts feel that it is associated with the tissues becoming sensitized as a result of previous low-grade bacterial infections. There also seems to be some hereditary connections to the disease. Stress and bad weather have also been implicated in recurrences of this condition.

Osteoarthritis is another very common form of chronic arthritis, but differs somewhat in its characteristics. It is more of a degenerative disease than an inflammatory one like rheumatoid arthritis. It affects both men and women, and more often occurs later in life. This form of arthritis tends to affect the larger weight bearing joints in the body, and is not usually bi-lateral in occurrence, possibly affecting only one joint at a time. It causes a degeneration of articular cartilages, with overgrowths of cartilage and bone, but does not generally cause a complete fusion of the joint. Also unlike rheumatoid arthritis, osteoarthritis is not usually accompanied by systemic reactions.

Although the exact cause of osteoarthritis is not known, it is thought to be associated with wear and tear on the body's joints, and often accompanies the aging process to some degree.

A hereditary form of arthritis, called **gout**, is a result of a metabolic problem with uric acid in the body. As a result, uric acid builds up in the bloodstream, and tends to precipitate out of solution and form urate crystals which accumulate in body tissues, especially around certain joints. Intense and painful inflammation of the joints may occur as acute attacks, often affecting the foot and knee areas. *(See Fig. 46)*

Bursitis is a condition involving inflammation of a bursa. Bursae are small, sac-like structures containing synovial fluid, and they function to reduce friction in areas where a lot of movement occurs, such as between tendons and bones around a joint.

Bursitis is often associated with a chronic irritation in the area, and commonly occurs in the shoulder and elbow regions. Bursitis in the elbow area is sometimes referred to as "tennis elbow".

Other Diseases of Bone

Osteoporosis is a term referring to the loss of bone density. Bone becomes more porous, brittle, and has a tendency to break more easily. Osteoporosis often accompanies old age to varying degrees, but is seen most commonly in women after menopause. Although the cause of osteoporosis is not exactly understood, it is known that gonadal hormones have an effect on the maintenance of bone tissue, and changes in these hormone levels can have adverse effects on bone.

Osteoporosis is also often seen in nutritional disorders, physical disuse such as in paralyzed patients, and other endocrine malfunctions.

Softening of bone tissue due to a loss of calcium is referred to as **osteomalacia** in adults and **rickets** in children.

Rickets is a childhood disease which occurs as a result of having a diet which is deficient in vitamin D. Vitamin D is necessary for the absorption of calcium from the digestive tract, and if it is not present in the diet in proper amounts, enough calcium cannot be absorbed for the body to use in the process of bone formation. Consequently, the bones of a growing child remain soft and deformed. This is especially noticeable in the long, weight bearing bones of the legs which may show a dramatic tendency to be bent or "bowed".

Osteomalacia may affect adults, but the effects are not usually as dramatic and severe as they are in a child, as ossification has already taken place in the adult body. Nevertheless, proper amounts of calcium are important in adults, as bones are dynamic organs, with a number of regular physiological activities occurring at all times.

Achondroplasia and **scoliosis** are examples of other developmental diseases affecting bones. Achondroplasia, which literally means "no cartilage formation", is a genetic disorder which results in a failure of cartilage to develop properly, especially in the growth centers of the long bones, resulting in a form of dwarfism.

Scoliosis is a condition in which the spinal column contains an abnormal lateral curvature. Although this condition is often a result of abnormal development, it may be an acquired problem as a result of disease involving other body structures, such as abnormally tilting hips, rickets, or disease of the muscles which function to hold the spinal column in its normal position.

Besides scoliosis, other abnormal curvatures of the spine may occur, either as congenital problems or as a result of such conditions as tuberculosis, rheumatoid arthritis, fractures, or tumors. **Kyphosis**, or "humpback", refers to an abnormal posterior curvature of the spine, while **lordosis** involves an exaggerated anterior curvature.

Tumors of bone and cartilage are also fairly common diseases. **Osteomas** and **chondromas** are benign tumors of bone and cartilage respectively, while the terms **osteosarcoma** and **chondrosarcoma** indicate malignancies of these tissues. Osteosarcomas are one of the most common forms of primary bone tumor, but bones are also a frequent site for the development of tumors which have metastasized from other areas in the body, such as carcinomas of the breast, lung, prostate gland, and the stomach. *(See Fig. 47)*

Fractures of bone are quite common, and are often sub-categorized based on additional detail about the nature and/or severity of the broken bone. Following are several examples of types of bone fractures:

1) compound fracture - one in which the broken bone pierces the skin, or an external wound leads down to the bone which is broken, such as in a gunshot wound

2) comminuted fracture - one in which bone is crushed or splintered into pieces

3) greenstick fracture - one in which the bone is bent on one side with a breakage on the opposite side, as would occur when one attempts to break a green stick

4) complete fracture - one in which two sections of bone are not touching, or completely separated from each other

Embalming Considerations

There are several embalming problems to be considered in reference to bone diseases. One of these is the problem created by fractures as a result of trauma. Certainly any bone is subject to fracture, but the more common ones to present difficulties for the embalmer are those of the skull and the extremities.

Fractures of cranial or facial bones can pose significant problems for the embalmer, as changes to the normal form and contour of these areas will accompany broken bones. Damage to these bones may require considerable reconstruction and wax modeling in order to restore a normal appearance. In addition, it should be anticipated that whenever facial or cranial fractures are encountered, swelling will also be a consideration, and care should be taken to avoid worsening the problem of swelling during arterial embalming by careful control of the injection pressure and rate of flow.

Fractures of bones in the extremities are also quite common, and may require the embalmer to straighten the affected limb as much as possible, and apply measures to hold the limb in the desired position for the completion of the embalming operation. This may include such steps as strapping or bandaging the broken limb, and even the application of a plaster of paris bandage after embalming in order to hold badly broken bones in position.

Bone procurement by anatomical donation agencies can also pose concerns for the embalmer. Entire bones, such as a femur, humerus, or os coxa, may have been removed for donation purposes. In these cases, it may be necessary for the embalmer to substitute some type of rigid material, such as a wooden dowel, to return a measure of rigidity to the affected area.

When bone procurement has been performed, the embalmer must also be aware that the vascular system in the area may have been compromised, and the use of additional injection points, or even hypodermic injection, for areas of the body beyond the procurement site may be necessary.

Inflammatory or degenerative diseases such as arthritis can also result in deformed and fused joints, making normal embalming and positioning of the body difficult. The embalmer may use such mechanical methods as stretching, massaging, and strapping into position of affected limbs in order to achieve desirable results. However, more extraordinary methods for straightening digits or limbs, such as incising tendons or the dislocation of joints, should not be attempted without written permission from survivors having the legal right to disposition.

Chapter Fourteen
DISEASES OF THE ENDOCRINE SYSTEM

Anatomy Review

The endocrine system is made up of those glands which release their chemical secretions directly into the blood. These secretions are referred to as hormones, and are delivered by the bloodstream to all parts of the body to chemically regulate many bodily functions. Because they do not have ducts, these glands are sometimes referred to as ductless glands, which differentiates them from exocrine glands, which have ducts to deliver their secretions to a specific body area. Glands which perform both endocrine and exocrine functions may be called heterocrine glands.

The secretion of different hormones into the bloodstream will have varying effects on the body. Some hormones are responsible for cellular metabolism in the body while others affect growth and development of the tissues. Other hormones have effects on such activities as sexual development or the concentration of substances such as salts or glucose in the bloodstream.

The main glands of the endocrine system include the pituitary, the thyroid, the parathyroids, and the adrenals. In addition, the pancreas and the sexual glands have both endocrine and exocrine functions, which qualifies them as examples of heterocrine glands.

Diseases of the Pituitary Gland

Located in the sella turcica of the sphenoid bone, and attached to the under surface of the brain, the pituitary gland is often referred to as the **master gland,** as a result of its far reaching effects in the body. Although it is small in size, measuring less than 1/2 inch in diameter and weighing approximately 1/60th of an ounce, it is very important in function. Appearing to be a single body, the pituitary is really two separate structures.

The anterior pituitary, or adenohypophysis, is responsible for the secretion of a number of hormones, including one called somatotropin, or growth hormone. This hormone stimulates the growth of bone and soft tissues in the body. Therefore, hypersecretion of this hormone in children, during the time they are actively growing, can result in a condition known as **giantism.** This condition of an abnormally tall person results from overstimulation of the growth process prior to ossification of the bones. Likewise, hyposecretion of this hormone during the growth years can result in a condition known as **dwarfism.** A person suffering from pituitary dwarfism is usually quite small, resembling a normally developed child, but does not develop secondary sexual characteristics.

If hypersecretion of somatotropin occurs in adults, after normal ossification and growth of the tissues has occurred, a condition called **acromegaly** results. While a person with this problem does not grow dramatically in height to become a giant, they do experience enlargement of many of the bones in the skull, hands, and feet. The facial features, including the nose, lips, and lower jaw, often thicken and become enlarged, resulting in a so-called "lion-faced" appearance.

Occasionally the pituitary gland of an adult becomes affected by such conditions as ischemic necrosis, or possibly a tumor, which results in a loss of pituitary function. This hypopituitarism in adults may be referred to as Simmond's disease, which is accompanied by a number of abnormal occurrences following diminished function of the body's "master gland". For example, **Simmond's disease** is characterized by emaciation, mental dullness, and general ill health. A person may experience premature aging, loss of sexual function, slow metabolism, and loss of body hair.

Diabetes insipidus, unrelated to the more common sugar diabetes, is a condition which involves the failure of the posterior lobe of the pituitary gland to secrete a proper amount of its hormone. This hormone is referred to as an anti-diuretic hormone because it controls the amount of water which is absorbed out of the urinary system back into the bloodstream. Without this hormone, excessive amounts of water are lost through the urinary system, causing serious dehydration of the body.

Diseases of the Thyroid Gland

The thyroid gland is located in the neck just below the larynx. Two large lobes separated by a narrow peninsula surround the trachea. The thyroid gland secretes a hormone called thyroxin which has regulatory control over general body metabolism. In essence, it controls the speed at which the cells of the body operate on a moment to moment basis. Because of this control exerted over the process of metabolism, the thyroid is a very important gland in proper development of many bodily functions.

When an excess of thyroid hormone is secreted, **hyperthyroidism** is said to occur. This condition occurs more frequently in females than in males. It is characterized by an increased metabolic rate, loss of weight, weakness, nervousness, and profuse sweating. **Grave's disease** is a special, and often severe, case of hyperthyroidism. In addition to the above mentioned symptoms, Grave's disease, also known as exophthalmic goiter, is characterized by bulging eyeballs due to edema of the tissues in the back of the eyesocket.

Hypothyroidism, which indicates a failure of the thyroid gland to produce sufficient hormone, can also have dramatic effects on both children and adults. When hypothyroidism is congenital, or occurs in the early years of life, it may be referred to as cretinism. Thyroxin is essential for proper development of the body, so an individual with cretinism remains a dwarf, both mentally and physically. Numerous disturbances are present in this condition, including mental retardation, poor development of bones, and failure of the sexual glands to develop.

If hypothyroidism occurs in adult life, the condition is referred to as **myxedema**. This condition is characterized by puffy skin due to infiltration of the tissues with a mucous-like edema. In addition, slow metabolism results in weight gain, mental dullness, and general sluggishness. Myxedema responds fairly well to administration of thyroid hormone, and dramatic improvements can be seen in a patient who has been effectively treated.

The term **goiter** is used to indicate an increase in the size of the thyroid gland. There are several different forms of goiter, which may be associated with various disorders of the thyroid, including hypersecretion, tumors, inflammations, and iodine deficiencies. Iodine is an important element used by the thyroid gland in forming thyroxin, and some cases of goiter are believed to be a form of compensatory hypertrophy caused by the body's demand for thyroxin when the diet is lacking in iodine.

Diseases of the Parathyroid Glands

The parathyroid glands secrete a hormone called parathormone, which has the effect of regulating blood calcium levels. Increased levels of parathormone, as a result of hyperparathyroidism, result in increased blood calcium levels. This increased level of calcium occurs because parathormone causes calcium to be drawn out of the bones and into the bloodstream. The condition often occurs as a result of tumor formation.

Calcium is an important element in the normal functioning of the body's cells, and the cells are sensitive to either too much or too little calcium. The excess calcium present in hyperparathyroidism can lead to various disorders in the body, including the **softening and deformation of bones**, formation of kidney stones, hardening of the arteries, and heartbeat irregularities.

When too little parathormone is produced, hypoparathyroidism exists, and blood calcium levels are likely to fall. Without enough calcium in the blood, nerve cells become irritable and overactive. This results in excessive stimulation of muscle cells by the nervous system, and can lead to abnormal, sustained muscle contractions called **tetany**.

Diseases of the Adrenal(Suprarenal) Glands

The adrenal glands are located on top of the kidneys. They consist of an outer layer called the cortex, and an inner layer called the medulla. The cortex of the adrenal glands, which is in turn under control of hormones from the pituitary gland, secretes several important hormones. These hormones help to regulate such conditions as salt levels in the blood, blood glucose concentration, and the production of some mild sex hormones. Consequently, malfunction of the adrenals can result in several different disease conditions, depending on which hormones are produced in abnormal amounts.

One common condition affecting the adrenal glands is referred to as **Cushing's syndrome**, which is a form of hyperadrenalism. If excess quantities of hormones called glucocorticoids are produced, as may happen due to a tumor of the gland, Cushing's syndrome can occur. It is characterized by greatly increased blood sugar levels, and also an increase in lipids or fats in the blood. A characteristic obesity usually occurs on the trunk of the body, resulting in the build-up of a fatty pad over the shoulders and upper back. Also, the face tends to become round and "moon-shaped". Patients with Cushing's syndrome also experience muscle weakness, fatigue, and high blood pressure.

Another form of hyperadrenalism occurs if there is an abnormal increase in the sex hormones produced by the adrenal cortex. Production of these hormones can result in a condition referred to as adrenogenital syndrome. This can lead to the pre-mature development of sexual characteristics in children, often referred to as sexual precociousness. If the condition occurs in females, they can experience the development of male secondary sex characteristics, such as a deepening of the voice and male distribution of body hair.

Hypoadrenalism occurs when a deficiency of certain adrenal hormones exists. One common form of hypoadrenalism is referred to as **Addison's disease**. The hormones which are involved in controlling water and salt levels in the body are primarily affected. There are digestive disturbances, low blood pressure, and the patient becomes dehydrated, emaciated, and generally weakened. The condition is also characterized by a deep brown or bronze discoloration of the skin due to these hormone imbalances.

Addison's disease can result from various conditions which destroy or cause atrophy of part or all of the adrenal gland. Such conditions may include infectious diseases like tuberculosis, neoplasms, and hemorrhage into the gland.

A condition called **Waterhouse-Friderichsen syndrome** is often discussed in connection with the adrenal glands, although it is actually a blood infection caused by the meningococcus organism. This is often a fulminating infection characterized by numerous hemorrhages into the skin, as well as severe adrenal hemorrhage, with rapid circulatory failure and death.

Diseases of the Pancreas

The pancreas is a heterocrine gland, meaning it performs both endocrine and exocrine functions. As its exocrine function the pancreas produces pancreatic juice, which is a digestive enzyme used for the breakdown of fats in the intestinal tract. As its endocrine function the gland produces two hormones, insulin and glucagon, which have regulatory control over the levels of glucose in the bloodstream.

Contained within the pancreas are patches of specialized cells called the Islets of Langerhans, and it is these cells which are responsible for producing the hormones insulin and glucagon. These hormones have antagonistic effects in the body, with insulin being responsible for lowering blood sugar levels, while glucagon raises the levels of glucose in the blood. When blood glucose levels fall, glucagon is secreted by the pancreas, which in turn stimulates the liver to release stored glucose into the blood for distribution to the cells of the body. When blood glucose levels rise, insulin is secreted, and it facilitates the movement of glucose out of the blood and into the cells.

Diabetes mellitus, often referred to as sugar diabetes, is a common disease condition which results from the failure of the pancreas to secrete proper amounts of insulin. This means that the sugars in the blood cannot be carried into the cells, and they tend to build up in the blood stream. The presence of excess sugars in the blood is referred to as **hyperglycemia**. Hyperglycemia then results in these excess sugars showing up in the urine, as there is more glucose present than the renal tubules of the kidney can absorb back into the bloodstream as they normally would. Excess sugar in the urine is called **glycosuria.**

Both hyperglycemia and glycosuria are considered important signs of diabetes mellitus. In addition, **polyuria**, or passage of excess quantities of urine, is also characteristic of diabetes, as the glucose in the blood acts as a diuretic, and additional water is needed to carry the glucose out of the body. Polyuria in turn can result in excessive thirst and dehydration.

When the cells of the body are deprived of their preferred nutrient, glucose, they begin to metabolize fats and proteins. This breakdown of fats results in a build-up of fatty acids in the blood, which can dramatically lower the ph level of the blood, a condition called acidosis. A significant lowering of the ph level of the blood can prove fatal if not corrected.

In addition to acidosis, the excess fats in the bloodstream predispose to atherosclerosis, or a fatty build-up on the inner lining of the blood vessels. Atherosclerosis then leads to occluded vessels and poor circulation. As you can imagine, poor circulation can lead to a variety of additional problems in the body, including the poor healing of wounds, which is another important complication of diabetes. This poor wound healing may be aggravated by the abnormal breakdown of tissue proteins, which can accompany the breakdown of fats in a diabetic patient.

The vascular obstruction associated with diabetes can have serious consequences, including myocardial infarctions, gangrene, and blindness due to ill effects on the capillaries in the retina of the eye.

There are different forms of diabetes mellitus, with the juvenile-onset type tending to be the most serious. It usually requires treatment with hypodermic injection of insulin, along with careful control of diet and exercise to balance the body's levels of glucose in the bloodstream. Adult onset diabetes may not be quite as serious, and may not require insulin injections, but close attention should still be paid to diet and exercise. Some oral medications are available to help the body use its supply of insulin in milder forms of diabetes.

Embalming Considerations

Many of the diseases we have discussed relative to the endocrine system can produce conditions which hamper the normal embalming operation.

Interference with normal circulation in the body is perhaps one of the most significant problems which can result from endocrine disorders, especially diabetes mellitus. The vascular obstruction which adversely affects normal life processes can also be a deterrent to adequate distribution of embalming fluid throughout the body. Careful control of injection pressure and rate of flow is necessary to achieve fluid distribution and tissue penetration without creating additional problems, such as swelling or hemorrhage. It is also likely that multiple injection sites will be required in any case involving vascular obstructions. Extreme cases such as those exhibiting gangrene of the extremities will require additional treatments, including hypodermic injection and surface compresses.

Edema is another post-mortem condition often associated with endocrine disorders, especially hypothyroidism. As with other cases of edema, close attention to the proper selection of arterial fluids should be a prime concern. The embalmer must anticipate that edematous cases will result in greater secondary dilution of arterial fluids, thus requiring the selection of a primary solution of adequate strength to sufficiently preserve the tissues.

Discolorations, such as those associated with Addison's disease, may also pose concerns for the embalming operator. Arterial fluids containing special dyes, such as jaundice fluids, may be helpful in overcoming these discolorations. In addition, dyes may be added separately to the arterial fluids of choice in order to obtain the desired effect. It is recommended that when dealing with such discolorations, the lower extremities be injected first so that the effects of the arterial fluids may be observed prior to injecting the head or upper extremities.

Various **deformities** such as those associated with dwarfism, or goiters which result from thyroid disorders, may also confront the embalmer. While these deformities will not necessarily require any special fluid considerations, they may require efforts to adjust, reposition, or reduce the deformity in order to achieve a more natural appearance. For example, it may be possible to reduce the size of a thyroid goiter with normal embalming procedures. However, if additional steps are deemed necessary, such as a major excision of tissues in order to achieve the reduction, written permission from the next of kin must be obtained.

Chapter Fifteen

DISEASES OF THE INTEGUMENTARY SYSTEM

Anatomy Review

The skin is the main organ of the integumentary system. It serves as a protective covering over the body, helps to regulate body temperature, and serves as an important sense organ for the body. Besides the skin itself, the integumentary system includes other structures often referred to as appendages to the skin. These include sweat and oil glands, sensory receptors, hair, and nails.

The primary outer layer of the skin is called the epidermis, which consists mainly of stratified squamous epithelium. Underneath the epidermis is the second primary layer of the skin, the dermis. The dermis is mainly connective tissue, and it supports many blood vessels, nerve endings, and other skin appendages.

Infectious Diseases of the Skin

Many infectious agents, including bacteria, fungi, viruses, and parasites are known to affect the skin. Some of these infections may be generalized, or systemic in nature, resulting in skin lesions which become apparent at various points during the course of the infection, or they may be localized, with the skin site being the primary portal of entry and focus of the organism causing the infection.

An abscess, which may be described as an area of pus surrounded by inflammatory tissue, is a lesion often found in the skin. It is commonly referred to as a **furuncle**, and it is usually the result of a local infection caused by the Staphylococcus aureus organism. When two or more furuncles join or communicate with each other, it may be referred to as a **carbuncle**.

Many other bacterial infections result in skin lesions at some point in their development. The secondary stage of **syphilis**, for example, is characterized by ulcerations on the mucous membranes, particularly in the mouth, and a reddish or copper colored skin rash. Tuberculosis of the skin, also known as **lupus vulgaris**, is characterized by patches or ulcerations which may leave scars on the skin after healing. **Scarlet fever**, which is a streptococcal infection characterized by sore throat, fever and other systemic symptoms, gets its name from the red skin rash which occurs during the disease.

Several genera of fungi often cause skin infections known as **dermatomycoses**, commonly referred to as "ringworm" or tinea. These include organisms from the genera *Microsporum, Trichophyton,* and *Epidermophyton.* These fungal infections have a tendency to localize in certain body areas, such as the scalp, beard, groin, or feet. Those affecting the groin area are sometimes referred to as tinea cruris, or "jock itch", and a fungal infection which often affects the feet, tinea pedis, is commonly called "athlete's foot". These infections are usually characterized by red, scaly, and itchy lesions, and may become further infected by bacteria if they are repeatedly scratched in an effort to relieve the itching.

Viruses are also well known for their ability to cause infection resulting in skin lesions. Examples of these viral diseases include:

1) measles (rubeola)

2) German measles (rubella)

3) Herpes simplex I - cold sores, fever blisters

4) Herpes simplex II - genital herpes, or venereal warts

5) Chicken pox (varicella) and shingles (herpes zoster)

6) Smallpox (variola)

These viral infections can result in varying forms of skin lesions, from the red spots of measles, to the pustular lesions of chickenpox, to the ulcerations and wart-like lesions of herpes infections.

Non-infectious Skin Diseases

Other forms of **dermatitis**, or inflammation of the skin, may result from non-infectious agents. Contact dermatitis, sometimes called **eczema**, results when the skin is exposed to agents to which it has become sensitized. Poison ivy or poison oak are good examples of skin irritations which result from contact with the resins of these plants, causing a blistering, itchy rash. Whether or not a certain individual contracts a case of poison ivy seems to involve a combination of the amount of plant resin they contact, plus their particular level of sensitivity to the allergen. Some individuals are not affected at all by contact with the resins of these plants.

Besides poison oak or poison ivy, numerous other chemical substances can result in contact dermatitis. Many products used in business and industry, such as soaps, lacquers, fabrics, dyes, formalin, and other chemicals have been known to cause cases of dermatitis.

Seborrheic dermatitis is a condition resulting from an excessive secretion of oil, called sebum, from the sebaceous glands in the skin, particularly the scalp area. It is a scientific term for what we might call chronic dandruff, and is characterized by a greasy and scaly scalp. This condition may spread to the face, neck, and eyebrow areas if not properly cared for.

Acne is another condition which results from an abnormal or profuse production of oil in the sebaceous glands. The pores of the skin often become clogged up with sebum, resulting in the production of pimples and blackheads. The condition commonly accompanies puberty to some degree, when increased hormone levels stimulate glandular activities in the body. Serious cases of acne can lead to permanent scars developing on the skin.

Tumors of various sorts routinely affect the skin, some of which are benign, and some are malignant. *(See Fig. 48)*

Papillomas are benign epithelial tumors which occur on the skin and mucous membranes. Those which develop on the skin, and are covered with a hard, rough layer of epithelium, are commonly referred to as warts.

Moles, or **nevi**, are pigmented epithelial tumors occurring on the skin. If moles enlarge dramatically in size, change color, bleed, or become painful, it may be a sign that they have turned cancerous, in which case they would be called **malignant melanomas**. Melanomas are highly malignant tumors, which can rapidly spread to other major organs in the body, and result in death if not properly treated in the early stages of development.

Squamous cell carcinoma and **basal cell carcinoma** are other examples of malignant forms of epithelial tumors affecting the skin. Carcinomas affecting the skin are most often associated with long-term, excessive exposure to the ultra-violet rays of the sun. *(See Fig. 49)*

Embalming Considerations

Various skin lesions routinely confront an embalmer and require special attention. Without going into a detailed listing of all possible skin lesions, it should be kept in mind that most such lesions will require additional treatment beyond routine arterial injection and venous drainage.

One category of post-mortem problems often encountered is **discolorations**. These discolorations may require hypodermic injection or surface compresses of bleaching agents in order to overcome the problem at hand. As a final method of dealing with skin discolorations, they may require an application of external cosmetics to achieve normal skin coloration.

Dehydration is a post-mortem condition which can result in dry and scaly skin. In addition to the use of the proper arterial fluids to counteract the effects of dehydration, surface treatment of dry skin can be of help in restoring natural appearance. Massage creams, and gentle scrubbing to remove scaly skin if necessary, can be quite beneficial in the embalming process.

Swelling may also accompany many skin conditions confronting the embalmer. Edema, hemorrhage under the skin, and various traumatic lesions predispose to swelling. These conditions should receive extra care, using accepted methods for the reduction of swelling in order to achieve desirable results in the embalming operation.

Various other skin conditions, such as ulcerations, burns, and pustular lesions, must receive special treatment in order to achieve the maximum degree of disinfection and preservation of tissues. Aspiration of pustular lesions, the use of surface compresses, and minor excisions of damaged, necrotic, or cancerous tissues may be necessary to effectively complete the embalming process. It should be mentioned, however, that any significant incision or excision of tissues beyond the normal, routine embalming operation, should be accomplished only after written permission is received from those with the right to disposition.

PATHOLOGY GLOSSARY

–A–

Abrasion - a superficial injury characterized by a scraping away of a portion of the skin or mucous membrane

Abscess - an area of pus surrounded by inflammatory tissue

Achondroplasia - a developmental disease characterized by the improper growth of cartilage in the long bones of the body, resulting in a form of dwarfism

Acne - an inflammatory disease of the skin and sebaceous glands, resulting in pustule formation and possible scarring

Acquired disease - any disease obtained after birth

Acromegaly - a condition characterized by enlargement and thickening of certain skull bones and facial features, as well as the bones of the extremities, due to hypersecretion of growth hormones by the pituitary gland after normal ossification has occurred

Acute disease - a disease of rapid onset and short duration

Active hyperemia - a form of hyperemia which results from the arterial system purposefully sending excess blood into a body part

Addison's disease - a disease resulting from hyposecretion of certain adrenal hormones, resulting in progressive weakness, emaciation, and a characteristic "bronzing" of the skin

Adhesion - an area of fibrous tissue holding two parts together which are normally separate, or unconnected

Albuminuria - the presence of an abnormal amount of serum albumin in the blood

Allergy - a state of hypersensitivity to foreign substances or allergens

Amelia - the congenital absence of one or more limbs

Amyloid disease - degeneration of organs or tissues as a result of the deposition of amyloid, a starch-like substance produced during certain metabolic disorders

Alzheimer's disease - a progressive, degenerative disease of the nervous system, resulting in memory loss, disorientation, and loss of various intellectual functions

Anasarca - generalized or widespread edema

Anemia - a decrease in the number of red blood cells and/or hemoglobin in the blood

Aneurysm - a localized weakening or dilation of an artery wall

Anomaly (malformation) - any abnormality of size, shape, or position of a body part

Anthracosis - discoloration of the lungs due to prolonged inhalation of coal dust ("black lung" disease)

Anuria - complete suppression of kidney function or urine formation

Aplasia - absence of a body part

Apoplexy - partial or total loss of brain function due to interruption of cerebral circulation as a result of hemorrhage, thrombosis, or embolism

Appendicitis - inflammation of the vermiform appendix

Arteritis - inflammation of an artery

Arteriosclerosis - disease of the arteries resulting in hardening, thickening, and loss of elasticity of the arterial walls

Arthritis - inflammation of a joint

Asthma - a form of allergy characterized by hypersecretion of mucous and spasms of the bronchial muscles, resulting in occluded air passageways

Ascites - edema of the abdominal (peritoneal) cavity

Asphyxia - a condition resulting from inadequate intake of oxygen

Atelectasis - a collapsed lung, resulting from pressure within the pleural cavity, or a blockage resulting in resorption of air from the alveoli

Atherosclerosis - a condition characterized by the build-up of fatty plaques on the inner lining of the arteries

Atrophy - a decrease in size of a body organ or part

Autopsy - examination of a dead body to determine the cause of death and/or the existence of pathological conditions; necropsy; post-mortem exam

Avulsion - forcible tearing away of tissue

–B–

Bronchitis - inflammation of the mucous membranes lining the bronchi

Bronchopneumonia - a form of pneumonia characterized by inflammation of the terminal bronchioles and alveoli

Bruise - an escape of blood into the subcutaneous tissue with discoloration but no broken skin

Bursitis - inflammation of a bursa

–C–

Calcification - infiltration and hardening of the tissues with calcium salts

Cancer - any malignant tumor

Carbuncle - inflammation of the subcutaneous tissues accompanied by suppuration and constitutional symptoms - may result from the joining of two or more furuncles

Carcinogen - any agent capable of causing cancer

Carcinoma - any malignant epithelial tumor

Cardiomyopathy - a general term referring to disease of the heart muscle

Caseation necrosis - the characteristic form of necrosis associated with tuberculosis, resembling a soft, cheesy mass

Cavitation - the formation of cavities within a tuberculous lung as a result of the necrotic material within a tubercle being sloughed off into an adjacent bronchiole

Cellular pathology (Microscopic pathology, Histo-pathology) - the study of disease based on observations made with the aid of a microscope

Cerebral palsy - non-progressive nervous system disorder characterized by brain damage before or shortly after birth, resulting in tremors, partial paralysis, and possibly mental retardation

Cerebrovascular accident (CVA) - changes in the brain which result from the interruption of cerebral circulation; also known as apoplexy or stroke

Cholangitis - inflammation of the bile ducts

Cholecystitis - inflammation of the gallbladder

Cholelithiasis - the process of gall stone formation

Chronic disease - one of relatively slow onset and long duration

Cicatrix - a scar left by a healed wound

Cirrhosis - chronic liver disease characterized by degeneration of the functioning liver cells and proliferation of connective tissue

Cleft palate - a congenital fissure in the roof of the mouth, forming a communicating passageway between the mouth and nasal cavity; may be accompanied by a cleft (hare) lip

Clinical pathology - that field of pathology dealing with the laboratory study of body fluids and secretions

Cold abscess - lesion resulting from the liquefaction of necrotic material in a tubercle; i.e., a chronic abscess containing pus, but without the signs of inflammation

Colitis - inflammation of the colon

Complication - any unfavorable condition which occurs during a disease

Communicable (contagious) disease - one which is easily transmittable from person to person

Concussion - disturbance of brain function, often temporary, as a result of a blow to the head

Congenital disease - a disease which is present at birth

Congestion - the accumulation of an excess amount of blood or tissue fluid in a body part

Contributory cause of death - the pathologic entity involved in but not causing the terminal event

Contusion - a bruise, often accompanied by swelling

Coryza - acute inflammation of the nasal mucous membranes, accompanied by profuse discharge; a common cold

Cretinism - congenital condition due to hypothyroidism in children, resulting in mental & physical retardation, including dwarfism

Creutzfeldt-Jakob disease - slow but progressive infectious disease of the nervous system, caused by a virus-like particle called a prion; causes an invariably fatal deterioration of the central nervous system

Cryptorchism (Cryptorchidism) - failure of the testes to properly descend into the scrotum

Cushing's Syndrome - a condition resulting from hypersecretion of glucocorticoids by the adrenal glands, resulting in obesity of the head and trunk, atherosclerosis, and hypertension

Cyanosis - bluish discoloration of the skin due to poorly oxygenated blood

Cyst - an abnormal, sac-like structure containing air, fluid, or a semi-solid substance

Cystic fibrosis - hereditary disease of exocrine glands, especially affecting the pancreas and respiratory system with occlusion, infections, and cyst formation

Cystitis - inflammation of the urinary bladder

–D–

Decubitus ulcer - localized area of necrosis on the skin, and progressing to the underlying tissues, due to prolonged external pressure over the area which cuts off the normal blood supply; a bed sore

Deficiency disease - a disease resulting from the lack of some essential element in body metabolism, such as the lack of a dietary vitamin

Degeneration - the deterioration of body cells/tissues with a corresponding loss of function

Dehydration - decrease in total body fluids

Diabetes insipidus - a condition characterized by polyuria as a result of a deficiency in anti-diuretic hormone being produced by the posterior lobe of the pituitary gland

Diabetes mellitus (sugar diabetes) - a condition characterized by the inadequate secretion of insulin by the pancreas, resulting in the failure of normal carbohydrate metabolism in the body

Diagnosis - the identification of a disease

Dilatation - dilation or expansion of an organ or vessel

Disease - the condition in which the structure and function of the body is impaired as a result of injury to the tissues; any abnormal structure or function occurring in the body

Diverticulosis - the presence of an abnormal sac or pouch in the walls of a hollow organ, such as the intestinal tract

Down's syndrome - a genetic disorder characterized by various degrees of mental retardation, a dwarfed physique, and other characteristic cranial and facial abnormalities

Dwarfism - condition of being abnormally small; pituitary dwarfism results from hyposecretion of growth hormone in children

Ecchymosis - a bruise on the skin as a result of hemorrhage into the subcutaneous tissues

Eclampsia - a condition associated with pregnancy, resulting in headaches, dizziness, nausea, and convulsions; often associated with pre-existing hypertension and glomerulonephritis

Ectopic pregnancy - implantation of a fertilized ovum outside of the uterus

Edema - an excess of tissue fluid in the intercellular spaces of the body

Emaciation - excessive weight loss or wasting away of the body

Embolism - obstruction of a blood vessel by a clot or any other substance which was carried to the point of obstruction by the bloodstream

Empyema - pus in the pleural cavity

Emphysema - overdistention, and often rupture, of the pulmonary alveoli

Encephalitis - inflammation of the brain

Encephalomalacia - softening of brain tissue

Endemic disease - one which is always present to some degree in a given area

Endocarditis - inflammation of the inner lining of the heart

Endocervicitis - inflammation of the lining of the cervix of the uterus

Endogenous pigmentation - discoloration of the tissues by normal body pigments

Endometriosis - the growth of endometrial tissue outside of the uterus, such as on the lining of the abdominal cavity

Endometritis - inflammation of the inner lining of the uterus

Enteritis - inflammation of the small intestine

Epidemic disease - one affecting a large number of people in the same area at one time

Epididymitis - inflammation of the epididymis

Epilepsy - a chronic nervous system disease characterized by sudden alterations in consciousness and frequently by convulsions

Epistaxis - bleeding from the nose

Erythrocytosis - an abnormal increase in the number of red blood cells

Esophagitis - inflammation of the esophagus

Etiology - the study of the causes of disease

Exacerbation - a sudden increase in the severity of a disease

Exciting factors - those factors involved in disease which are directly responsible for causing the disease; immediate factors

Exogenous pigmentation - discoloration of the tissues due to pigments which entered the body from the outside

Exudate - fluid which collects around an inflammation site; serous exudates contain much fluid, hemorrhagic exudates contain blood, and purulent exudates contain pus

–F–

Febrile disease - one characterized by fever

Fistula - an abnormal channel or passageway through the tissues connecting an organ with an internal body cavity or with the surface of the body

Forensic pathology - the field of pathology involving both the medical and legal aspects surrounding death; medico-legal pathology

Fulminating disease - one of severe and sudden onset, which often proves fatal

Functional disease - one which does not show recognizable lesions

Furuncle - an abscess located in the deeper layers of the skin, as in a hair follicle

–G–

Gangrene - necrosis of tissues due to a lack of blood supply; may be called dry gangrene if bacteria are absent, or moist gangrene if it turns putrefactive by the invasion of saprophytic bacteria

Gas gangrene - necrosis and putrefaction of tissue as a result of the invasion by a gas producing bacillus, especially *Clostridium perfringens*

Gastritis - inflammation of the stomach

General pathology - that field of pathology dealing with widespread processes such as necrosis, inflammation, and degeneration, without regard to individual body organs or systems

General paresis - degeneration of brain tissue seen in tertiary syphilis

Giantism - condition resulting from hypersecretion of pituitary growth hormone in children

Gingivitis - inflammation of the gums

Glomerulonephritis - a form of nephritis, or kidney inflammation, affecting the capillary structures within the kidney

Glossitis - inflammation of the tongue

Glycosuria - excess sugar in the urine, often associated with diabetes mellitus

Goiter - enlargement of the thyroid gland

Gout - a form of arthritis resulting from the build-up of uric acid in the blood and leading to the formation of urate crystals in and around joints; an hereditary metabolic disorder

Grand mal - a severe form of epilepsy characterized by convulsions and loss of consciousness

Grave's disease - a condition characterized by increased metabolism, weight loss, and nervousness as a result of hypersecretion of thyroid hormone

Gross Pathology - field of pathology which involves the study of changes in the structure and function of the body which may be observed with the unaided eye

Harelip - congenital malformation of the upper lip resulting from improper fusion of tissues during the developmental process

Hay fever - form of allergy characterized by irritation of the upper respiratory passages and eyes caused by the pollen of various plants

Hematemesis - bleeding from the stomach; also known as blood in the vomit

Hematoma - a localized tumor-like swelling filled with blood, as in a blood blister

Hematuria - whole blood in the urine

Hemoglobinuria - the presence of hemoglobin in the urine

Hemophilia - hereditary bleeding disorder characterized by an abnormal tendency to bleed as a result of a genetic disorder in the blood clotting mechanism

Hemoptysis - blood in the sputum; bleeding from the lungs or upper respiratory tract

Hemorrhage - escape of blood from the vascular system

Hemorrhoids - varicose veins of the rectum or anal area

Hemothorax - bleeding into the pleural cavity

Hepatitis - inflammation of the liver

Hereditary disease - a disease which is passed on from parents to offspring as a result of a genetic defect

Hernia - protrusion of an organ through the walls of the body cavity which contains it

Histo-pathology - the field of pathology dealing with changes in structure and function of the tissues which are observed with the aid of a microscope; cellular pathology; microscopic pathology

Hydrocele - collection of edematous fluid in a sac-like cavity in the body, most commonly edema of the scrotum

Hydrocephalus - excessive collection of cerebrospinal fluid within the ventricles of the brain, causing compression of the brain and possibly enlargement of the cranium

Hydronephrosis - the build-up of urine in the kidney pelvis as a result of an obstruction to the outflow of the urine

Hydropericardium - the collection of edematous fluid in the pericardial cavity

Hydrothorax - collection of edematous fluid in the pleural cavity

Hyperemia - excess blood in a body part; congestion

Hyperglycemia - excess sugar in the blood

Hyperplasia - an increase in the size of a body part due to an increase in the number of cells in that part

Hypertension - high blood pressure

Hypertrophy - increase in the size of a body part due to an increase in the size of the cells in that part

Hypoplasia - incomplete development of a body part

–I–

Iatrogenic disorder - any adverse condition induced in a patient as a result of the effects of a treatment given by a doctor

Incompetence - failure of a damaged valve to operate properly; insufficiency

Idiopathic disease - a disease of unknown cause

Immediate factors - those factors involved in disease which are directly responsible for causing the disease; exciting factors

Infarction - death of tissue due to a lack of blood supply

Infection - the invasion of the body by pathogens which cause injurious effects; inflammation caused by living agents

Infectious disease - a disease caused by pathogenic microorganisms

Infestation - the presence in or on the body of macroscopic organisms, such as lice or fleas

Infiltration - the passage and accumulation of a substance into cells, tissues, or organs

Intoxicating disease - a disease caused by a poisonous or toxic substance

Intussusception - a slipping or "telescoping" of one section of intestine into an adjacent section

Intracranial hemorrhage - hemorrhage within the cranial cavity

Ischemia - decreased blood flow to a body part

–J–

Jaundice - yellowish discoloration of the tissues due to the presence of bile pigments (bilirubin) in the blood; icterus

–K–

Kyphosis - "humpback" or abnormal posterior curvature of the spine

–L–

Laceration - a tearing of the tissues

Laryngitis - inflammation of the larynx or voice box

Lesion - an area of structural damage as the result of disease

Leukemia - a malignancy of the hemopoietic tissues, characterized by a massive increase in the number of white blood cells present in the body

Leukocytosis - an increase in the number of white blood cells

Leukopenia - a decrease in the number of white blood cells

Liquefaction necrosis - necrotic material which has taken on a liquid state, as may happen within a tubercle in tuberculosis

Lobar pneumonia - a form of pneumonia which tends to be consolidated in one or two lobes of the lung(s)

Lordosis - abnormal anterior curvature of the spine

Lymphangitis - inflammation of lymph vessels

Lymphedema - edema due to obstruction of lymphatic vessels

Lymphoma - a malignancy of the lymphoid tissues in the body, such as in Hodgkin's disease

–M–

Malformation - a defect or anomaly

Medico-legal pathology - that field of pathology involving the legal and the medical issues surrounding death; forensic pathology

Meningitis - inflammation of the meninges

Metaplasia - conversion of one type of tissue into another type which is not normally present at that location, but within the same general category, such as one form of epithelial tissue changing into another type of epithelial tissue

Metastasis - the spread of tumor cells from one location to another via the blood or lymph streams

Metritis - inflammation of the uterus; uteritis

Microscopic pathology - that field of pathology dealing with changes in the structure and function of the tissues which may be observed with the aid of a microscope; cellular pathology; histo-pathology

Miliary tuberculosis - form of tuberculosis where the lesions are scattered widely in various body organs and tissues

Multiple sclerosis - degenerative disease of the nervous system characterized by the formation of plaques on nerve cells which in turn impairs their normal control functions of body parts

Myelitis - inflammation of the spinal cord

Myocarditis - inflammation of the heart muscle

Myxedema - a condition characterized by puffy skin, weight gain, and general sluggishness as a result of hypothyroidism

–N–

Necropsy - a post-mortem examination of the body; autopsy

Necrosis - a localized area of dead tissue

Neoplasm - any new, abnormal growth of tissue which serves no useful purpose in the body; tumor

Nephritis - inflammation of the kidney

Nephrolith - a kidney stone; renal calculus

Nephrolithiasis - the process of kidney stone formation

Nephrosis - non-inflammatory degenerative disease within the kidney

Neuritis - inflammation of a nerve

Nevus - a pigmented, generally benign tumor of the skin; mole

Nosocomial infection - one acquired in a hospital or health care facility

–O–

Occlusion - blockage of an opening or passageway

Occupational disease - a disease related to one's working conditions

Oligemia - less than the normal amount of blood in the body

Oliguria - passage of less than the normal amount of urine

Oncology - the study of tumors

Oophoritis - inflammation of the ovaries

Orchitis - inflammation of the testes

Organic disease - a disease characterized by recognizable lesions

Osteitis - inflammation of a bone

Osteomalacia - abnormal softening of the bones in adults

Osteomyelitis - inflammation of the bone marrow

Osteoporosis - disease of bone characterized by the loss of bone density and increased porosity

–P–

Paget's disease - skeletal disease of the elderly, with chronic bone inflammation resulting in thickened and softened bones

Pancreatitis - inflammation of the pancreas

Pandemic disease - a disease which is epidemic in many areas at the same time, possibly world-wide

Papilloma - an epithelial tumor often appearing on the skin, with a hardened surface; a wart

Passive hyperemia - excess blood in a body part due to a blockage in the venous return of blood

Parkinson's disease - a chronic, degenerative nervous system disorder, characterized by tremors, muscle weakness, and a peculiar gait; "shaking palsy"

Pathogen - any organism capable of causing disease

Pathogenesis - the origin and development of a disease

Pathological anatomy - the study of structural changes present during disease; morbid anatomy

Pathology - the science dealing with the study of disease

Pericarditis - inflammation of the pericardium

Peritonitis - inflammation of the peritoneum

Petechiae - small spot-like, or "pin-point", hemorrhages in the skin or mucous membranes

Petite mal - a mild form of epilepsy

Pharyngitis - inflammation of the pharynx, or throat

Phlebitis - inflammation of a vein

Phocomelia - a congenital condition in which the proximal portions of the limbs are poorly developed or absent

Physiological pathology - the study of functional changes in the body as a result of disease

Pigmentation - the passage or accumulation of abnormal amounts of coloring matters into the tissues

Plethora - an increase in total blood volume in the body

Pleural effusion - the accumulation of edematous fluid in the pleural cavity; hydrothorax

Pleuritis - inflammation of the pleura; pleurisy

Pneumoconiosis - infiltration of the lungs with various forms of dust

Pneumonia - inflammation of the lungs; pneumonitis

Pneumothorax - air in the pleural cavity

Poliomyelitis - inflammation of the gray matter in the spinal cord as a result of a viral infection

Polycythemia - an increase in red blood cells; erythrocytosis

Polydactylism - an excess number of fingers or toes

Polyp - a "stalked" or stemmed tumor growing from the mucous membranes especially the nasal and intestinal areas

Polyuria - the passage of excess quantities of urine

Post-mortem examination - the examination of the body after death; necropsy; autopsy

Pre-disposing factors - those factors involved in disease which make it more likely one will contract a disease, but don't actually cause the disease

Proctitis - inflammation of the rectum

Prognosis - a prediction of the probable outcome of a disease

Prostatitis - inflammation of the prostate gland

Purpura - purplish discoloration of the tissues due to widespread hemorrhages into the skin or mucous membranes

Pustule - a small elevation on the skin containing pus; pimple

Pyelitis - inflammation of the kidney pelvis

Pyelonephritis - inflammation of the kidney and the kidney pelvis

Pyothorax - the presence of pus in the pleural cavity; empyema

Pyuria - the presence of pus in the urine

–R–

Recurrent disease - a disease which has a tendency to return at intervals; it shows alternating increases and decreases in its symptoms

Regeneration - replacement of damaged cells with identical cells

Remission - a let-up in the severity of a disease

Renal calculus - a kidney stone; nephrolith

Repair - literally to replace or heal, but often used to indicate replacement of damaged tissue with connective tissue, as opposed to regeneration

Resolution - the termination of an inflammatory reaction

Rheumatic fever - a disease which can cause damage to the heart and other organs as a result of an allergic reaction to a previous streptococcal infection such as tonsillitis

Rhinitis - inflammation of the nasal mucous membranes

Rickets - a deficiency disease of children, resulting from a lack of vitamin D in the diet, which causes improper calcification of bones, which in turn leads to soft and malformed bones

–S–

Salpingitis - inflammation of the fallopian tubes

Sarcoma - a malignancy of non-epithelial tissue

Seborrheic dermatitis - excessive secretion of oil from sebaceous glands, often in the scalp, resulting in a greasy, scaly skin

Scoliosis - abnormal lateral curvature of the spine

Sebaceous cyst - a cyst filled with oil from a distended sebaceous gland in the skin

Shock - a state of collapse, characterized by depressed vital signs and possibly unconsciousness, as a result of circulatory failure; often accompanies hemorrhage, trauma, burns, and other serious conditions

Sign - an objective indication of the presence of disease, such as heat, redness, or swelling

Silicosis - infiltration of the lungs with stone dust

Simmond's disease - hypopituitarism in adults, resulting in premature aging and general ill health

Sinusitis - inflammation of the paranasal sinuses

Special pathology - that field of pathology which deals with diseases affecting particular body organs or systems

Splenomegaly - enlargement of the spleen

Spina bifida - a congenital defect in which the inferior portion of the spinal column fails to properly form, resulting in a herniation of the contents of the spinal cavity; congenital fissure of the spinal column

Sporadic disease - a disease which occurs occasionally in a given area

Stenosis - abnormal narrowing of an opening or passageway; stricture

Stomatitis - inflammation of the mouth

Stroke - partial or total loss of brain function due to interruption of cerebral circulation as a result of hemorrhage, thrombosis, or embolism

Suppuration - the process of pus formation

Surgical pathology - the field of pathology which deals with the study of tissues removed from the body during surgery

Symptom - a subjective indication of the presence of disease, such as pain, itching, or nausea

Syndrome - a group of signs or symptoms

Syphilis - infectious venereal disease caused by *Treponema pallidum*

–T–

Tabes dorsalis - degeneration of the posterior part of the spinal cord as a result of tertiary syphilis

Thrombocytopenia - a decrease in the number of circulating platelets in the bloodstream

Thrombosis - the formation of a blood clot within the cardiovascular system

Transient ischemic attack (TIA) - temporary interference with the blood supply to the brain

Tracheitis - inflammation of the trachea

Tubal pregnancy - implantation and development of a fertilized ovum in the fallopian tube

Tubercle - the lesion of tuberculosis

–U–

Ulcer - an area of localized necrosis on the skin or mucous membrane

Uremia - the presence of toxic waste products in the bloodstream as a result of a diseased kidney failing to perform its filtering function

Ureteritis - inflammation of the ureter(s)

Urethritis - inflammation of the urethra

–V–

Vaginitis - inflammation of the vagina

Varicocele - varicose veins of the spermatic cord

Varicose vein - a vein which is abnormally dilated and tortuous

Vesicle - an elevation on the skin containing fluid, as in a blister

Volvulus - a twisting of a segment of intestine

–W–

Waterhouse-Friderichsen syndrome - a severe, often fulminating, meningococcal blood infection which results in adrenal hemorrhage

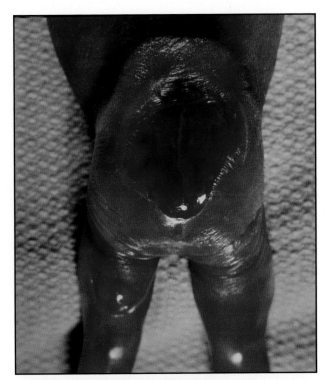

FIG. 1 – Spina Bifida

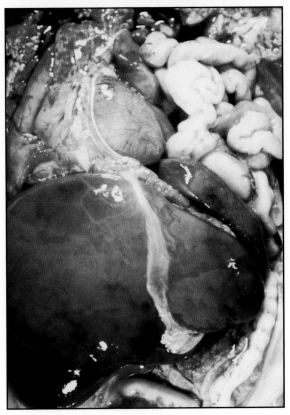

FIG. 2 – Severe diaphragmatic hernia
(Note intestines protruding into the thoracic cavity)

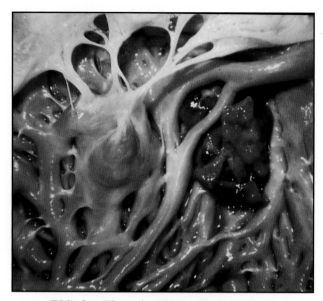

FIG. 3 – Thrombus located in the heart

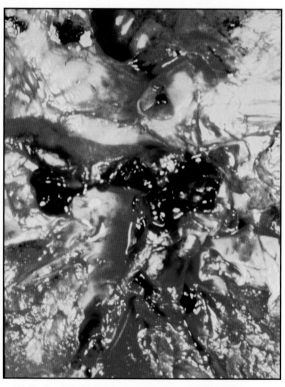

FIG. 4 – Pulmonary embolism (Dark areas)

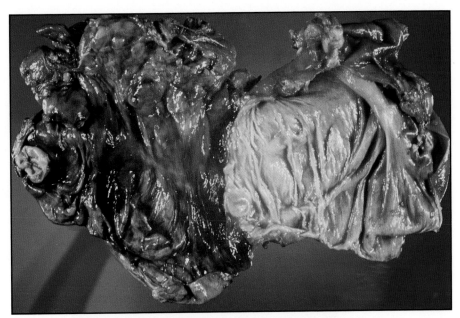

FIG. 5 – Ischemic necrosis of the intestine (Dark area)

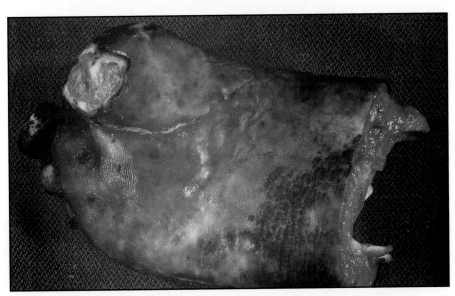

FIG. 6 – True gangrene of the foot, resulting in amputation

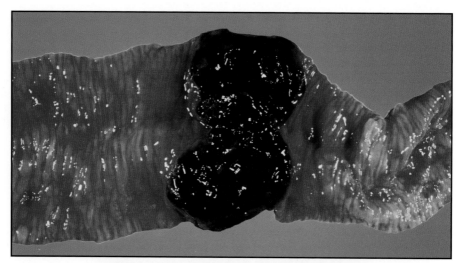

FIG. 7 – Hemotoma in the small intestine

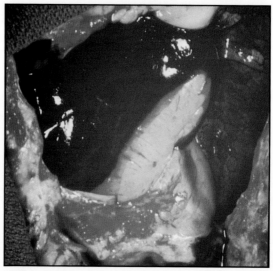

FIG. 8 – Hemopericardium
(Note: Hemopericardium is the dark area above the heart.)

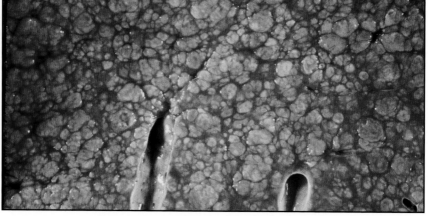

FIG. 9 – Fatty degeneration of the liver

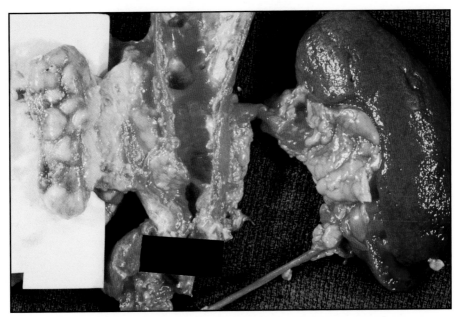

FIG. 10 – Atrophied kidney due to renal artery stenosis

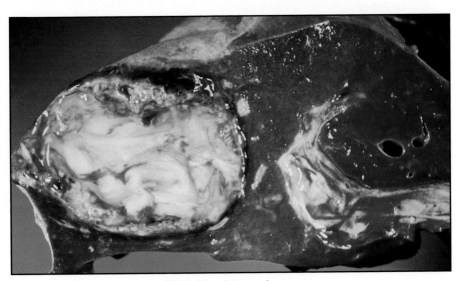

FIG. 11 – Liver abscess

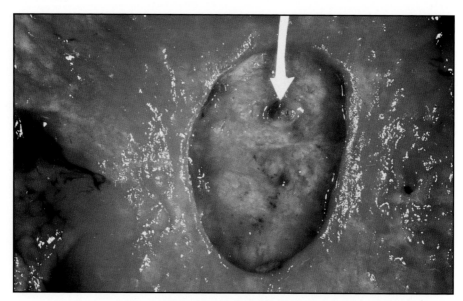

FIG. 12 – Stomach ulcer

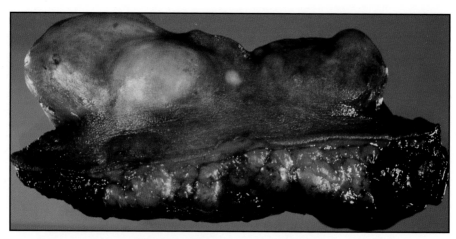

FIG. 13 – Fibrosarcoma of the skin

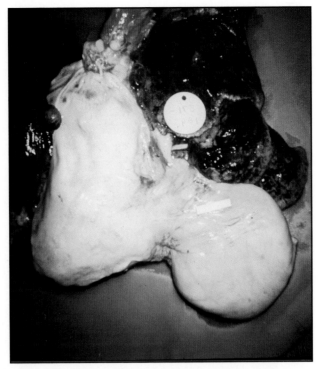

*FIG. 14 – Large lipoma affecting the pericardium
(lower right area of photo, shown from a posterior view)*

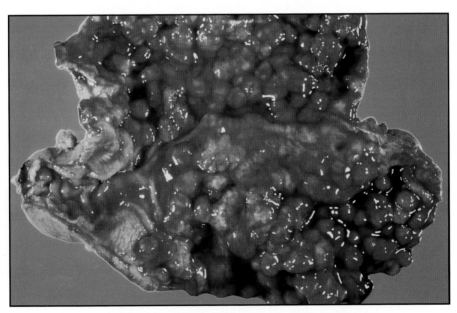

FIG. 15 – Multiple polyps in the stomach

115

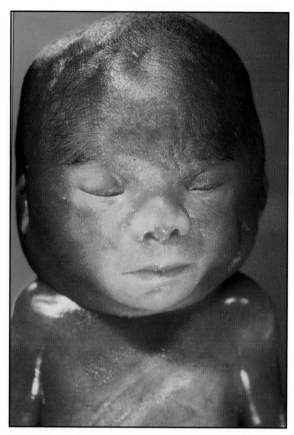

FIG. 16 – Edematous fetus as a result of liver and circulatory failure after erythroblastosis fetalis

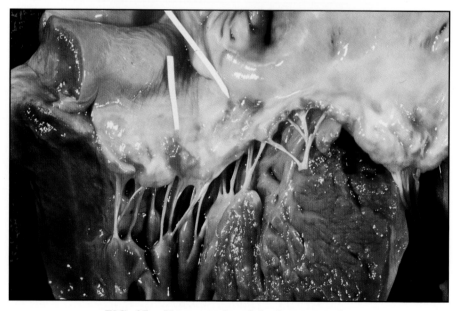

FIG. 17 – Hypertrophy of the heart muscle, also showing valvular lesions from endocarditis

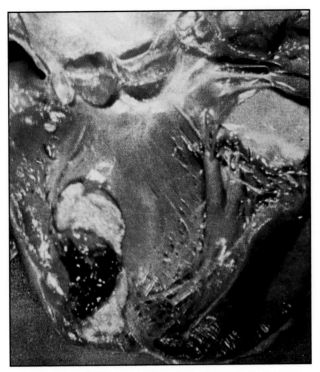

*FIG. 18 – Heart thrombus (dark area) on top of
infarcted myocardium (light area)*

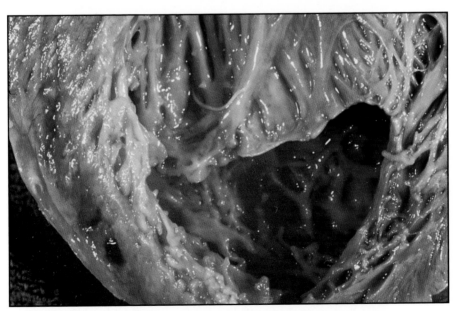

*FIG. 19 – Myocardial infarction (dark area on left side)
and ruptured interventricular septum*

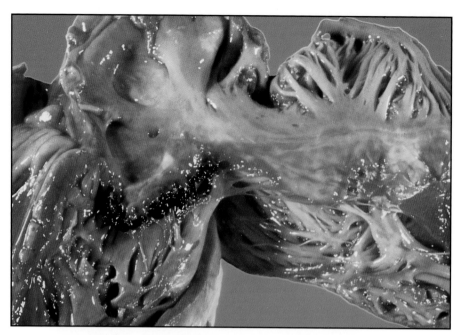

*FIG. 20 – Endocarditis showing vegetative lesions
on the atrioventricular valve*

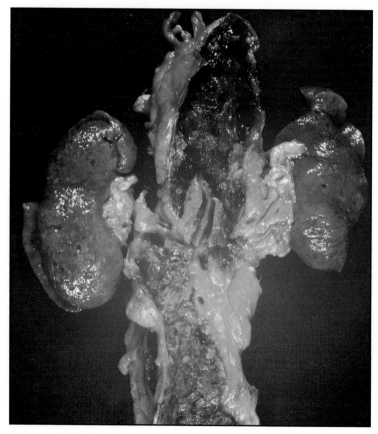

*FIG. 21 – Thrombosis (darker area at top) and
atherosclerosis in the abdominal aorta*

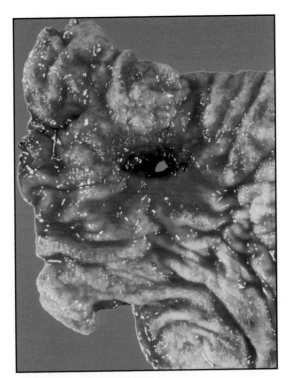

FIG. 22 – Perforated stomach ulcer

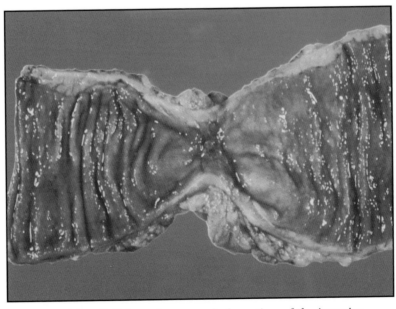

FIG. 23 – Colitis, stricture and ulceration of the intestine

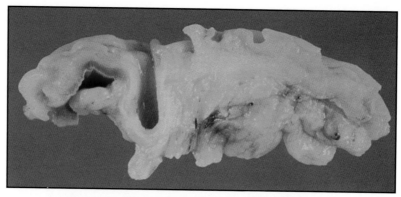

FIG. 24 – Diverticulum in the wall of the colon

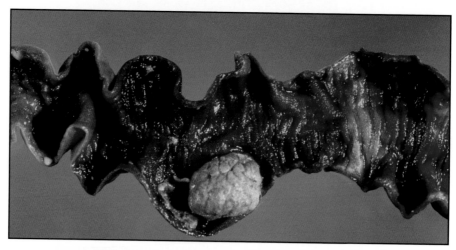

FIG. 25 – Intussusception of the small intestine
(shown with large clump of bacterial growth in affected area

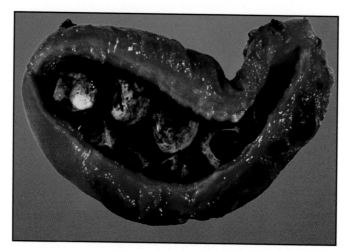

FIG. 26 – Multiple gallstones in the gallbladder

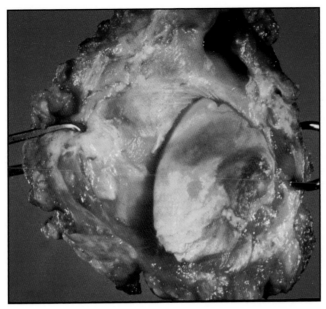

FIG. 27 – Large gallstone in the gallbladder

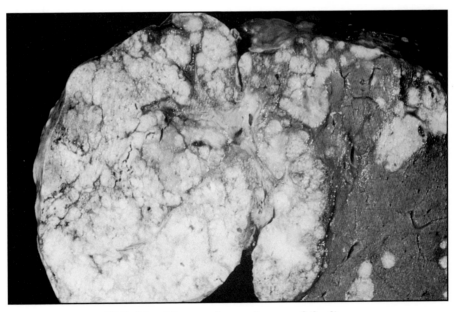

FIG. 28 – Metastatic carcinoma of the liver

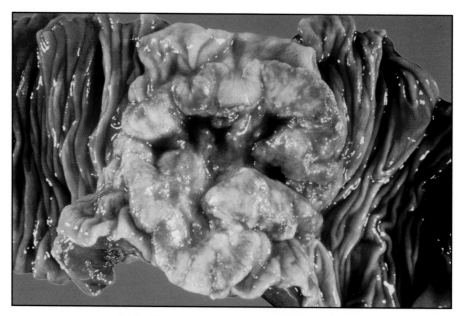

FIG. 29 – Adenocarcinoma of the colon

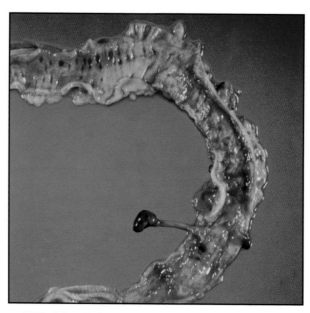

FIG. 30 – Polyp and diverticulosis of the colon

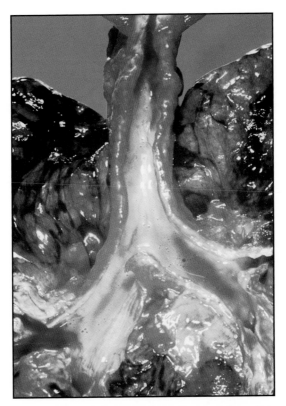

FIG. 31 – Bronchitis (dark area along the margins of the bronchi)

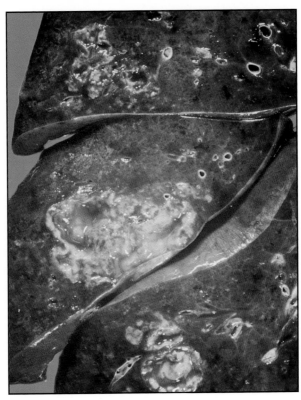

FIG. 32 – Bronchopneumonia with abscess formation

123

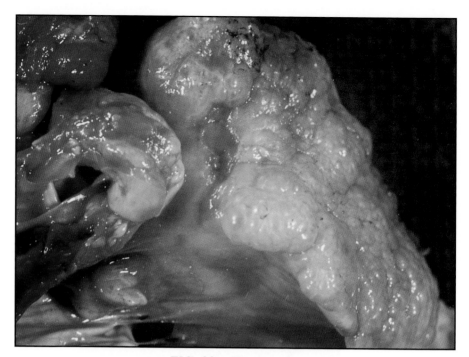

FIG. 33 – Emphysema

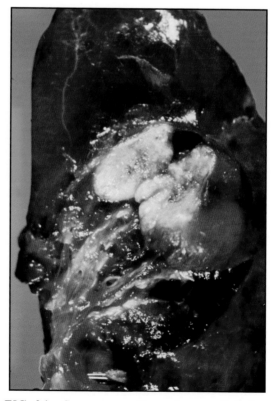

FIG. 34 – Squamous cell carcinoma of the lung

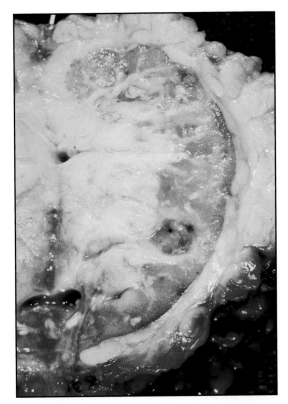

FIG. 35 – Pyelonephritis (light areas in the center)

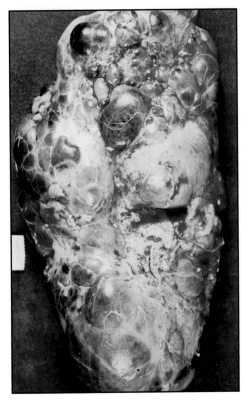

FIG. 36 – Polycystic Kidney

125

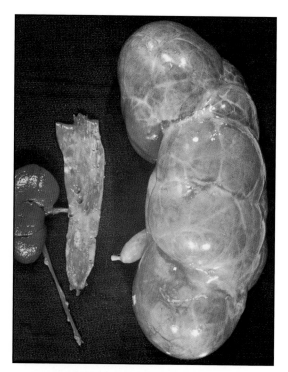

FIG. 37 – Severe hydronephrosis

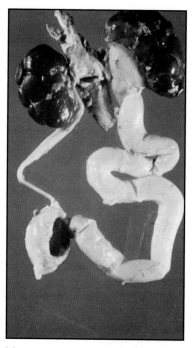

FIG. 38 – Hydronephrosis and hydroureter

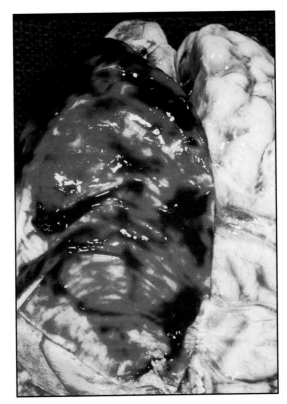

FIG. 39 – Sub-dural hematoma

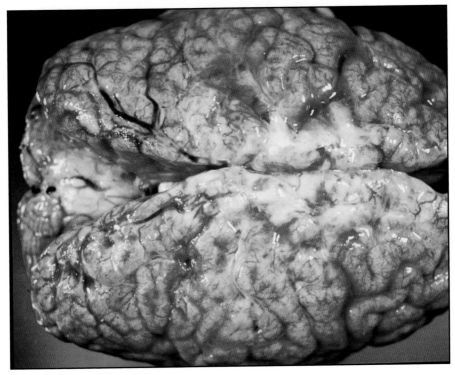

FIG. 40 – Purulent meningitis

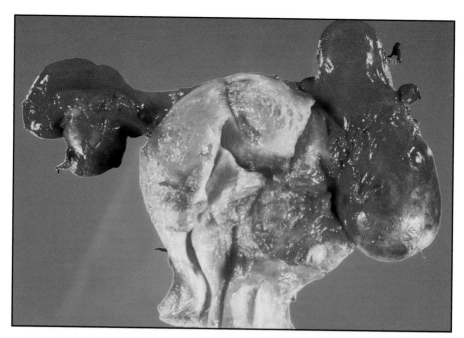

FIG. 41 – Tubal/ovarian abscess (right side of picture)

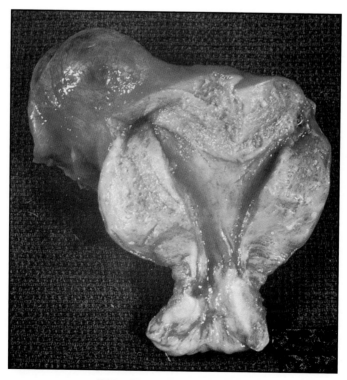

FIG. 42– Tubal pregnancy

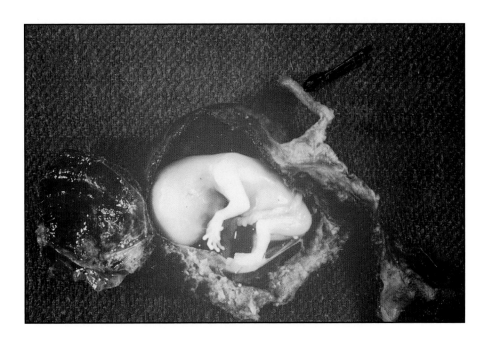

FIG. 43 – Tubal pregnancy

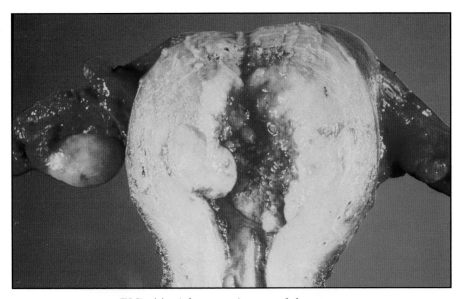

FIG. 44– Adenocarcinoma of the uterus

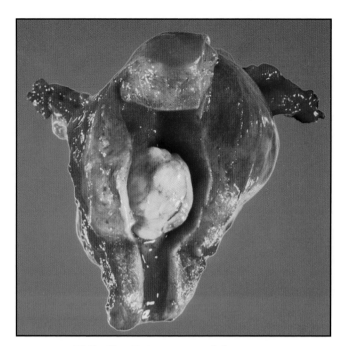

FIG. 45 – Leiomyoma of the uterus

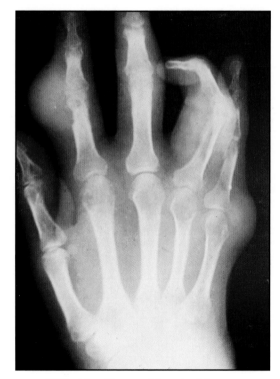

FIG. 46 – X-ray of hand with gout

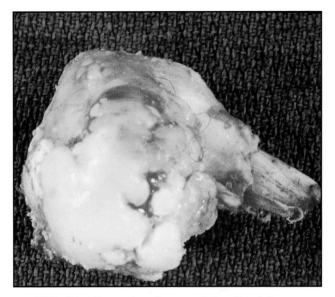

FIG.47 – Osteochondroma of the distal femur

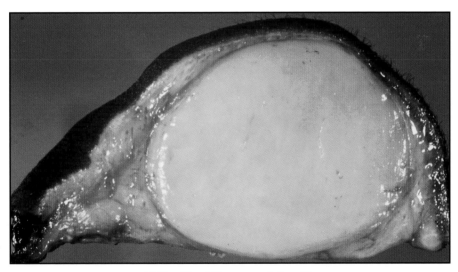

FIG. 48 – Fibroma of the skin

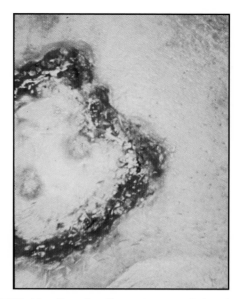

FIG.49 – Basal cell carcinoma of the skin